Eating Disorders

Eating Disorders

L. K. George Hsu

THE GUILFORD PRESS
New York   London

*To my wife, and to the
memory of my parents.*

© 1990 The Guilford Press
A Division of Guilford Publications, Inc.
72 Spring Street, New York, NY 10012

Printed in the United States of America

This book is printed on acid-free paper.

Last digit is print number: 9 8 7 6 5 4 3 2

Library of Congress Cataloging-in-Publication Data

Hsu, L. K. George (Lee Keung George)
    Eating disorders / L. K. George Hsu.
        p.   cm.
    Includes bibliographical references.
    ISBN 0-89862-401-0
    1. Eating disorders.   I. Title.
    [DNLM: 1. Eating Disorders.   WM 175 H873e]
RC552.E18H78   1990
616.85′26—dc20
DNLM/DLC
for Library of Congress   89-17179
                                                    CIP

Preface

This book is written to provide, in a single volume, a summary of the current knowledge on the eating disorders of anorexia nervosa and bulimia nervosa. While it necessarily reflects some personal views, I have nevertheless presented my understanding of these intriguing disorders in the context of a review of the current literature. It is not, however, an exhaustive review. Instead, I have focused primarily on conceptual and empirical findings in the field that I consider to be of interest to clinicians, particularly those who treat adolescent patients, and to academics who are interested in a convenient summary of such issues. I have therefore included some biomedical material that may be less comprehensible to those without a medical background, because I believe that an understanding of these aspects is essential to the daily practice of the clinician and because I believe they hold promise for further advances in the field. I have not included much psychodynamic material, not because I am opposed to it, but because empirical data on psychodynamic research are not available. While I do not hold the reductionist view that a scientific approach is all-sufficient for an understanding of the eating disorders, and I need not remind my readers that the very assumptions on which empirical research is based are themselves outside the realm of scientific methods, I nevertheless believe that clinicians and academics, and of course the patients, stand to gain the most from better empirical research. Therefore, to the extent that this book stands between multi-author volumes covering many aspects of the eating disorders on the one hand and rather idiosyncratic single-author monographs on the other, I believe that it fills a gap in the literature by presenting a coherent review and synthesis of the current thinking and findings on these disorders.

Chapter 1 outlines the historical development of the concepts of anorexia nervosa and bulimia nervosa; it also discusses the identity of the disorders with respect to their relationships to each other, to simple dieting, and to the affective disorders. It therefore sets forth my own view on the nature of these disorders. Chapter 2 describes the clinical features of the disorders and includes, among other issues, a discussion of why I do not accept the idea that there is a disturbance of body image in the eating disorders. Chapter 3 reviews the epidemiology of the disorders, from which I conclude that simple dieting and the eating disorders occur on a behavioral continuum. In Chapter 4, I review the etiological findings and present my view that dieting provides the entrée into an eating disorder if it was intensified by certain adolescent issues and accompanied by the presence of certain risk factors. This explains why the disorders are more common, for instance, among females than males and in developed than developing countries. In Chapter 5, I describe the diagnostic evaluation process, with particular reference to the adolescent patient, and discuss the current diagnostic criteria of the disorders. I also defend my adoption of both the continuous and the categorical model in my formulation of the concept of these disorders. Chapter 6 describes the treatments of these disorders, again with particular reference to the adolescent patient. I advocate the adoption of a flexible, eclectic approach guided by common sense and available empirical data. In Chapter 7, I review the outcome of the disorders. A knowledge of outcome is important in that it provides us with the proper perspective with which to view our treatment efforts. I also discuss the nosology of the disorders in the light of the outcome data. In the Epilogue, I briefly summarize my views on the primary prevention and future research of the eating disorders.

Throughout this book, I have used feminine pronouns to refer to the patients in an effort to avoid grammatical awkwardness and to reflect the predominance of the eating disorders among females.

This book was written in the midst of great personal turmoil and could not have come to be without the support of my family, and the many individuals who have helped on both a professional and personal level to make this task possible. To all of them I owe my deep and sincere gratitude. The following list is but a very partial one of these individuals. First and foremost, I am indebted to my many teachers, in particular Arthur Crisp, who have taught me about the eating disorders, and among them I count all my patients. Second, I am most appreciative to my "team" for their unfailing assistance and support: Beth Fryman, Robin Santhouse, Lisa Clement, Betty Chesler, Dianne Deep, Theresa Sobkiewicz, and Georgette Connor. They have sustained me with their clinical acumen and infectious enthusiasm, and this book reflects their contributions toward my understanding of the eating disorders. Third, I thank Tom Ollendick and David Garner for their careful review of earlier drafts of this book. Fourth, I thank my friend Tom Burns for his hospitality, support, and encouragement during my recent stay in London when this book was going through its final stages of rewriting. Last but not least, I thank Seymour Weingarten, my editor at Guilford, for his willingness to publish this volume and for his encouragement and advice throughout this project.

Contents

1

Conceptualizing the Eating Disorders

The eating disorders of anorexia nervosa (*anorexia* is from the Greek for "loss of appetite") and bulimia nervosa (*bulimia* is from the Greek for "ox appetite") are characterized by an implacable and distorted attitude toward weight, eating, and fatness. The illnesses usually begin in adolescence and carry considerable morbidity and mortality. The apparent increase in their incidence recently and the interest they have generated both within the scientific community and among the general public have created the impression that these are novel diseases of our times. However, although scientific writings on the two disorders were uncommon before the early 1960s, the eating disorders are by no means recent discoveries. The term *anorexia nervosa* was first used by Sir William Withey Gull (1816-1890), a physician at Guy's Hospital in London, in a paper published in 1874 in which he described the case histories of four women, including one for whom the illness was fatal. He had first mentioned the illness briefly, calling it apepsia hysterica, in a lengthy address on diagnosis in medicine that he delivered in Oxford in 1868 (Gull, 1874). However, by 1874, he felt that "anorexia would be more correct" (p. 25), and he preferred "the more general term 'nervosa,' since the disease occurs in males as well

1

as females" (pp. 25–26). He emphasized as part of the clinical picture of the illness the presence of amenorrhea, constipation, bradycardia, loss of appetite, emaciation, and in some cases low body temperature, edema of legs, and cyanotic peripheries. He commented particularly on the remarkable restlessness and "mental perversity" of the patients and was convinced that the loss of appetite was "central" in origin. He found the illness to occur mainly in young females between the ages of 16 and 23.

Ernest Charles Lasegue (1816–1883), a professor of clinical medicine in Paris, published an article, "De l'Anorexie Hysterique," in 1873 in which he reported on eight patients. He found the illness to occur mostly in young women between the ages of 15 and 20, with the onset precipitated by some emotional upset. He also described the occurrence of diminished food intake, constipation, increased activity, amenorrhea, and the patient's contentment with her condition despite the entreaties and threats of family members.

Many early accounts of what might have been the condition of anorexia nervosa are available (for a review, see Bliss & Branch, 1960). The clearest and most detailed account is probably the treatise by Richard Morton, a London physician, in his *Phthisiologia: Or a Treatise of Consumptions,* first published in Latin in 1694. In the book he described several conditions of consumption, devoting one section to the condition of "nervous consumption" in which the emaciation occurred without any remarkable fever, cough, or shortness of breath. He believed the illness to be the result of "violent passions of the mind, the intemperant drinking of spirituous liquors, and an unwholesome air" (quoted in Bliss & Branch, 1960, p. 60). He then described two cases, an 18-year-old woman who subsequently died following a "fainting fit" and a 16-year-old boy who made a partial recovery. Despite these promising beginnings, the concept of anorexia nervosa was not clearly established until our own time. The main reason for the conceptual confusion was the overgeneralized interpretation of the nature of the patient's refusal to eat. A second source of confusion was the erroneous view that severe emaciation was a frequent, if not cardinal, feature of hypopituitarism, a condtion first described by Simmonds in 1914. That anorexia nervosa was not related to hypopituitarism was finally clarified by Sheehan and Summers in 1949, but the overgeneralized interpretation of the nature of the food refusal persisted into the early 1960s. Thus, for instance, in an otherwise exceptionally comprehensive account of anorexia nervosa, Bliss and Branch (1960) nevertheless chose to define anorexia nervosa as simply "a malnutrition due to deficient diet, in which the caloric restriction is entirely psychological" (p. 24). Similarly, in one of the earliest psychiatric studies of anorexia nervosa, Kay and Leigh (1954) concluded categorically that "the psychiatric symptomatology is diverse. . . . We are not convinced that we have been dealing with a psychiatric entity" (p. 428). However, in all fairness, most of the cases that Bliss and Branch and Kay and Leigh described would probably have qualified for primary anorexia nervosa according to our present criteria.

If anorexia is taken to mean a loss of the desire to eat, then there is no doubt that the term *anorexia nervosa* is a misnomer. It is indeed unfortunate that even the Feighner criteria (Feighner et al., 1972) use the term *anorexia* without defining or clarifying its meaning. The anorectic patient refuses to eat not because she has no appetite, but because she is afraid to eat; the food refusal or aversion to eating is the result of an implacable and distorted attitude toward weight, shape, and fatness. The idea that this characteristic attitude is the cardinal feature of the disorder was not clearly formulated until the early 1960s by investigators such as Bruch (1966), who described this feature as a "relentless pursuit of thinness" (p. 555), while Crisp (1967) described it as a "weight phobia" (p. 5), and Russell (1970) as "a morbid fear of becoming fat" (p. 134). Once this concept took hold, the illness of anorexia nervosa became distinguishable from other illnesses that led to similar malnutrition. Thus, for instance, a person with hysteria may refuse to eat because of somatic complaints, such as an inability to swallow, and a depressed patient may refuse to eat because of a genuine loss of appetite, but neither demonstrates the characteristic "relentless pursuit of thinness." More recently, however, there has been a revival of the idea that the eating disorders are merely variants of an affective illness, an issue that is discussed later in this chapter.

Occurrences of vomiting and binge eating in the context of anorexia nervosa were clearly described by Bliss and Branch (1960) and Meyer (1961). Later, Beumont, George, and Smart (1976) proposed that there are two subgroups of anorectic patients: the restrictors and the vomiters. This idea was taken further by both Casper, Eckert, Halmi, Goldberg, and Davis (1980) and Garfinkel, Moldofsky, and Garner (1980), who divided anorexia nervosa into the restrictor and the bulimic subgroups. The occurrence of binge eating in the context of obesity was described as early as 1959 by Stunkard, and in 1970 Kornhaber described the condition as the "stuffing syndrome." Meanwhile, Nogami and Yabana (1977) in Japan proposed that kibarashigui (binge eating with an orgiastic quality) be delineated as a separate syndrome from anorexia nervosa. The confusion produced by using a symptom (bulimia) to describe a syndrome (also bulimia) is considerable, and in the English-speaking world the terms *bulimarexia* (Boskind-Lodahl & White, 1978), *dietary chaos syndrome* (Palmer, 1979), *bulimia nervosa* (Russell, 1979), and *abnormal normal weight control syndrome* (Crisp, 1979) have been proposed for the binge-eating syndrome in patients with a normal or near-normal weight. In 1980 the *DSM-III* (APA, 1980) distinguished *bulimia* as a syndrome from anorexia nervosa, and in 1987 the *DSM-III-R* (APA, 1987) changed the term to *bulimia nervosa*. Despite the fact that the attempt to delineate bulimia nervosa from anorexia nervosa is relatively recent, clinical descriptions of what appeared to be the disorder were published by Pierre Janet in 1903 (see Pope, Hudson, & Mialet 1985) and perhaps as early as 1767 by Robert Whytt (see Bliss & Branch, 1960), who described a 14-year-old boy who, having lost weight through anorexia, suddenly began to "have such a craving for food with a quick digestion that he grew faint unless he ate every two hours" (p. 12).

However, doubts still persist regarding the identity of the eating disorders. On the one hand, the boundary between the disorders and "normal" dieting behavior seems blurred. On the other, the eating disorders are sometimes considered to be variants of other psychiatric illnesses, previously schizophrenia and obsessive–compulsive disorder, more recently the mood disorders. The discussion of the identity of the eating disorders is not entirely academic; in order for research on the disorders to continue, investigators have to agree on a definition of the disorders so that they are distinguishable from, say, a major depression or from each other. In essence, the discussion amounts to defining a concept that makes the most sense. In this chapter, I review the distinction between anorexia nervosa and normal dieting, anorexia nervosa and bulimia nervosa, and the eating disorders and other psychiatric disorders, in particular the affective disorders. Some of these ideas are discussed in greater detail in subsequent chapters.

DIETING AND THE EATING DISORDERS

Because so many of the symptoms and behaviors of an anorectic patient occur as the result of dieting to lose weight, could it be argued that anorexia nervosa is simply dieting that has gotten out of hand? Epidemiological studies clearly demonstrate that the population group that is most concerned about dieting and weight is also the one with the highest incidence of the disorder (see Chapter 3). Further, in nonclinical populations many individuals show a subclinical form of the disorder (Button & Whitehouse, 1981; Nylander, 1971; Patton, 1988b; Szmukler, Eisler, Gillis, & Hayward, 1985); that is, although they demonstrate many or all of the features of the disorder, their symptoms do not meet the researchers' severity criteria (e.g., they might not have lost 25% of their premorbid weight and thus did not qualify for one of the diagnostic criteria). The fact that amount of weight loss is used as a criterion implies some continuity between dieting and the disorder of anorexia nervosa. Many "recovered" anorectics still demonstrate excessive preoccupation with weight and dieting, much as "normal" dieters would. Finally, the terms *fear of fatness* and *pursuit of thinness* suggest that the phenomenon is quantitative rather than qualitative.

The answer to our question lies partially in how one conceptualizes the disorder. Bruch (1973), for instance, conceptualized anorexia nervosa as the "desperate struggle for a self-respecting identity" (p. 250) and described three areas of disordered psychological functioning: a disturbance of delusional proportions in body image and body concept, a disturbance in the accuracy of the perception or cognitive interpretation of stimuli arising in the body, and a paralyzing sense of ineffectiveness. Arguing that anorectics are actually afraid of being at a normal weight rather than being overweight, Crisp (1967, 1980) conceptualized anorexia nervosa as a psychologically adaptive stance operating within biological mechanisms, a weight-based phobic avoidance posture stemming from a fear of the demands of a normal adolescent/adult body weight; in short, a psychobiological regression from adolescence. Both Bruch and Crisp believed that the motivation of the anorectic to go on a diet is fundamentally different from that of the average teenager.

In an attempt to clarify the continuity/discontinuity issue, Garner, Olmsted, Polivy, and Garfinkel (1984) used the Eating Disorder Inventory (EDI) to study three groups of females: college students, ballet students, and anorectic patients. Women in the first two groups were divided into weight-preoccupied and non-weight-preoccupied subgroups on the basis of their dieting and weight concern as reflected by scores on the Drive for Thinness subscale of the EDI. The researchers found that relatively few of the weight-preoccupied women scored above the anorectic median on three of the EDI subscales: Ineffectiveness, Interpersonal Distrust, and Lack of Interoceptive Awareness. Using cluster analysis procedures, they were able to divide the weight-preoccupied women into two subgroups: one showing elevated scores on all the EDI subscales and one best described as normal dieters. The authors concluded that while some dieters may superficially resemble anorectic patients in their pursuit of thinness, they do not in fact show the other central psychopathological features of anorectic patients (e.g., sense of ineffectiveness and interpersonal distrust). While these findings are intriguing and deserve further investigation, this study fails to show clearly that the EDI scores of the weight-preoccupied group and the anorectic group are indeed discontinuous; that is, there is no bimodal distribution of scores on any of the subscales. Further, the study raises our original question of whether the group of weight-preoccupied women with high EDI scores should be given the diagnosis of subclinical anorexia nervosa. Finally, it has not been demonstrated that the weight-preoccupied "normal" dieters do not, in time, develop an eating disorder. In fact, available evidence indicates that adolescent dieters are much more likely to develop an eating disorder than their nondieting counterparts (see Chapter 3). Thus, perhaps the question is not whether anorexia nervosa is qualitatively distinct from normal dieting, but rather what factors turn the latter into the former.

In Chapters 3 and 4, I develop the view that eating disturbances ranging from simple dieting to diagnosable eating disorders occur on a behavioral continuum and that dieting provides the entrée into an eating disorder if it was intensified by certain adolescent issues and accompanied by certain risk factors. However, in taking this position I also recognize that patients with diagnosable eating disorders demonstrate certain features quantitatively and perhaps also qualitatively different from those that occur in normal dieters. I discuss this "categorical" (i.e., caseness) versus "continuum" (i.e., dimensional) issue further in Chapter 5. Suffice it to say here that extreme deviations from the mean on any psychopathological dimension (in this case, dieting behavior) are also associated with a higher probability for "caseness," which in turn is identifiable by certain associated features (e.g., fear of fatness) related in varying degrees to the particular dimension in question. Later in this chapter I speculate on the nature of the fear of fatness, a cardinal feature of the disorders.

THE DISTINCTION BETWEEN ANOREXIA NERVOSA AND BULIMIA NERVOSA

The distinction between anorexia nervosa and bulimia nervosa is by no means clear-cut unless we use body weight as a distinguishing feature. Bruch (1985) refused to accept that normal-weight bulimia was either a clinical entity or related to primary anorexia nervosa, although she readily acknowledged that bulimia and vomiting could occur in anorexia nervosa (Bruch, 1973). However, investigators have found that many restrictive anorectics in time may develop the syndrome of normal-weight bulimia nervosa (e.g., Bruch 1985; Crisp, Hsu, Harding, & Hartshorn, 1980), while some 50% of normal-weight bulimics give a definite history of anorexia nervosa (Hsu & Holder, 1986; Lacey, 1983; Russell, 1979). Russell (1985) and Lacey (1983) proposed that bulimia nervosa be diagnosed only in those with a previous history of anorexia nervosa. Although disagreeing with this view (see Chapter 5), I concede readily that the distinction between the two conditions is blurred. Recent studies have shown that in some respects the bulimic anorectic resembles more closely the normal-weight bulimic than her restricting counterpart (Garner, Garfinkel, & O'Shaughnessy, 1985). For instance, the bulimic anorectic demonstrates more impulse dyscontrol behavior, such as stealing and using street drugs and alcohol, and on certain psychometric tests the bulimic anorectic scores much more like the normal-weight bulimic than the restrictive anorectic. Family studies of anorectics (Strober, Morrell, Burroughs, Salkin, & Jacobs, 1985) indicated that increased rates of anorexia nervosa, bulimia nervosa, and subclinical anorexia nervosa occurred among their first- and second-degree relatives compared to normal controls. This pattern of familial clustering suggests that these disorders may represent variable expressions of a common underlying psychopathology. However, the sevenfold increase in the risk of bulimia with or without anorexia nervosa in female relatives of bulimic anorectics compared to restrictive anorectics also suggests that bulimia may be transmitted separately and specifically. There is also evidence that restrictive anorexia nervosa, bulimic anorexia nervosa, and normal-weight bulimia nervosa all run true-to-form (see Chapter 7). Finally, I believe it is confusing to give an emaciated anorectic with occasional bulimic episodes the same diagnosis as a normal-weight or overweight bulimic patient, since the management of these patients is quite different. I therefore believe that before all the evidence is in, it is heuristically more meaningful to retain the more traditional subdivision of anorexia nervosa into the restrictive and vomiter/bulimic groups, confining bulimia nervosa to those with a normal or near-normal body weight. The classification of the eating disorders is discussed further in Chapter 5.

THE EATING DISORDERS
AND OTHER PSYCHIATRIC ILLNESSES

As already mentioned, there have been many attempts historically to link anorexia nervosa to other psychiatric disorders. Brill (1939), for instance, was struck by the withdrawn and "schizoid" features of the patients, and regarded anorexia nervosa as a forme fruste of schizophrenia. Nicolle (1938) shared this view, and even Bruch (1964) at one point felt that there was a link between anorexia nervosa and schizophrenia on account of the patients' perceptual disturbances. To my knowledge, no one has recently suggested that anorexia nervosa may be a form of schizophrenia. Other investigators have focused on the obsessive–compulsive features of the disorder, in particular the preoccupation with food and weight, as well as the compulsive behavior concerned with eating and exercise, and have suggested that anorexia nervosa may be related to an obsessive–compulsive disorder (e.g., Palmer & Jones, 1939; Rahman, Richardson, & Ripley, 1939). Dally (1969) subdivided anorectics into an obsessive group, a hysterical group, and a group with mixed obsessive and hysterical features. Recently, some interest in this linkage has been revived (e.g., Rothenberg, 1986). In particular, since there is intense speculation that disturbances in the serotonin neurotransmitter system may be related to the development of anorexia nervosa (e.g., Morley & Blundell, 1988) and since there is mounting evidence that disturbances in the same neurotransmitter system occur in obsessive–compulsive disorder (Zohar, Insel, Zohar-Kadocuh, Hill, & Murphy, 1988), a link at the neurochemical level between the two disorders is possible. In my view, however, it would be premature at this stage of our knowledge of the neurotransmitters to suggest that anorexia nervosa is a variant of obsessive–compulsive disorder.

It is the issue of whether the eating disorders are variants of an affective illness that has generated the most debate (e.g., Altshuter & Weiner, 1985; Pope & Hudson, 1988; Strober & Katz, 1987). Many early authors have commented on the depression frequently experienced by anorectic patients (e.g., Fenichel, 1945; Nemiah, 1950), and some have even suggested that anorexia nervosa may be a form of suicide (e.g., Brill, 1939), or a compromise with it (Crighton-Miller, 1938). Several findings are relatively incontrovertible. Eating-disorder patients often complain of feeling sad or at least look dejected, and they often suffer from poor self-esteem and are socially and emotionally withdrawn. Perhaps as many as 60% of patients cross-sectionally meet criteria for depression in structured interviews (Bentovim, Marilov, & Crisp, 1979; Cooper & Fairburn, 1986; Herzog, 1984; Walsh, Roose, Glassman, Gladis, & Sadik, 1985); and on rating scales or self-report measures (Eckert, Goldberg, Halmi, Casper, & Davis, 1982; Hsu & Crisp, 1980; Lee, Rush, & Mitchell, 1985; Swift, Kalin, Wamboldt, Kaslow, & Ritholz, 1985). Cantwell and colleagues (Cantwell, Sturzenberger, Burroughs, Salkin, & Green, 1977) suggested that anorectics on follow-up tend not to suffer from anorexia nervosa but instead develop a major depression. Most family studies indicate that there is an increase in the prevalence of affective illness in the biological first- and second-degree relatives of patients with eating disorders (see Chapter 2, section on Family Characteristics). Certain biological findings, such as the activation of the hypothalamic–pituitary–adrenal axis, that occur in affective disorders also occur in the eating disorders (see Chapter 2, section on Endocrine Disturbances). Finally, bulimic, although not anorectic, patients may respond well to antidepressants (see Chapter 6).

However, despite the evidence from these five areas (similarity in clinical features, possible "transformation" of anorexia nervosa to affective disorder, higher prevalence of affective illness in relatives of eating-disorder patients, similar biological disturbances, and similar treatment response to antidepressants), the relationship between the two disorders is far from being straightforward. The clinical picture of depression in eating-disorder patients is mixed, with perhaps less than one-third meeting strict criteria for major depression (Bentovim et al., 1979; Walsh et al., 1985). In those patients with a dual diagnosis of an eating disorder and an affective disorder, the two disorders do not always share the same time of onset (Piran, Kennedy, Garfinkle, & Owens, 1985; Walsh et al., 1985). Furthermore, the symptoms of the eating disorder and the affective disorder do not always covary; remission or exacerbation of one may bear no temporal relationship to that of the other (Hsu, 1980; Swift et al., 1985). The course and outcome of anorexia nervosa (Hsu, 1980) and bulimia nervosa (Swift, Ritholz, Kalin, & Kaslow, 1987) bear no obvious resemblance to those of affective disorders (Keller, 1985). For affective disorders, two-thirds of patients are recovered from the index episode at 6 months after presentation for treatment, whereas the rates of recovery from anorexia nervosa and bulimia nervosa at 6 months are probably much lower. The most common diagnosis of patients who have recovered from anorexia nervosa (i.e., regained normal weight) is bulimia nervosa, not major depression (see Chapter 7). Strober and Katz (1987) suggest that depression might represent a final common pathway for many chronic psychiatric disorders not genetically related to one another, such as alcoholism, antisocial personality disorder, schizophrenia, and the eating disorders. If confirmed, this may explain why dysphoria is so common among eating-disorder patients at follow-up. The severe malnutrition of anorexia nervosa readily produces multiple biochemical and endocrinological disturbances (for a review, see Halmi, 1980; Isaacs, 1979), and despite their relatively normal body weight, bulimic patients likewise suffer from malnutrition (Pirke, Pahl, Schweiger, & Warnhoff, 1985). While there is some evidence to suggest that a few disturbances may persist in anorectics despite apparent weight recovery, such as an abnormal glucose tolerance (Crisp, Ellis, & Lowry, 1967) and elevated corticotropin-releasing hormone (Kaye et al., 1987), the significance of these findings remains unclear. On balance, the evidence does not support the view that the eating disorders are variants of affective illnesses. I find the linkage of anorexia and bulimia nervosa to, say, the affective illnesses to be important not so much in indicating that they may be variants of one another but for suggesting the possibility that therein lie some mechanisms that turn normal dieting into anorexia nervosa or bulimia nervosa. In Chapter 4, I will present my speculation that a person who is predisposed to develop an affective illness is more likely to develop an eating disorder if she goes on a diet.

THE IDENTITY OF THE EATING DISORDERS

It is interesting that although anorectics and perhaps also bulimics are struggling for a sense of personal identity, psychiatrists are arguing over the identity of the eating disorders themselves. Kay and Leigh (1954) stated emphatically that "there is no neurosis specific to anorexia nervosa and no specific anorexia nervosa" (p. 431). Many later authors concurred with this view (Lesser, Asheden, Debriskey, & Eisenberg, 1960; Seidensticker & Tzagournis, 1968; Warren, 1968). Russell (1970), in arguing for a separate identity for anorexia nervosa, suggested that there are three criteria by which to judge whether a disorder deserves to be given a separate identity; (1) whether there is a constancy of association of the various clinical features; (2) whether there is similarity in the course and outcome of the illness and, especially, whether the illness "breeds true"; and (3) whether a clear-cut etiology has been elucidated.

The evidence that anorexia nervosa has a consistent nucleus of clinical features is overwhelming. Intermediate and long-term outcome studies, which are reviewed in Chapter 7, also amply support the view that the illness breeds true. While the long-term outcome of bulimia nervosa is unknown, intermediate (4-6 year) follow-up studies suggest that it also runs true-to-form (see Chapter 7). The elucidation of a clear-cut etiology for the eating disorders remains an unfulfilled objective, but this is the case for most of the other psychiatric disorders. Kendell (1975) has therefore argued that the delineation of a psychiatric disorder should be based on "the criterion of discontinuity" of symptoms from those of its neighbor. Attempts to delineate other psychiatric syndromes have, however, yielded mixed results. For instance, the issue of whether endogenous depression is distinct from neurotic depression, or whether depressive illness is distinct from anxiety disorder, is still unsettled (Kendell, 1969; Post, 1972). There is currently very little empirical data from which to build a system of diagnostic categories, and, as we have mentioned, the decision often hinges on which concept makes the most sense.

It is my conviction that the central and cardinal feature of the eating disorders is the distorted attitude toward weight, eating, and fatness that breeds the characteristic fear of fatness. As such, they stand apart from other illnesses that do not share this feature. This disturbance persists in patients even at follow-up, and the fact that both anorexia nervosa and bulimia nervosa run true-to-form strongly suggests that these disorders should be regarded as distinct diagnostic categories.

However, ultimately the important question may not be whether the eating disorders are distinct entities, but what lessons they can teach us regarding the interplay between cultural, interpersonal, intrapsychic, and biological forces and factors. As we shall see in Chapters 2 and 3, the disorders most commonly affect young Caucasian females from the middle to upper social classes in developed countries. Since the same population is also most commonly engaged in dieting and other weight-control behaviors, sociocultural factors are clearly involved. Further, the fact that the illnesses almost always have their onset in adolescence suggests that certain developmental processes may have become deranged. Finally, the presence of a family history of affective illnesses suggests that certain biological or psychological vulnerability may predispose the dieting individual to develop an eating disorder.

The intriguing feature for anorexia nervosa is the finding that the fear of fatness actually intensifies as the individual loses weight, while for bulimia nervosa the fear is accompanied by an irresistible urge to binge and purge. There is no satisfactory explanation for the occurrence of this fear of fatness. It does not seem to qualify as a delusion, and most eating-disorder patients do not demonstrate any other psychotic features. In an intuitive leap, Bruch (1962) linked it with a disturbance of body image. This apparent conceptual breakthrough has generated much research in body-size perception and bodily attitudes and affect. However, as we shall summarize in Chapter 2, body-size perceptual distortion does not represent body-image disturbance and is not pathognomonic of the eating disorders. Elsewhere I have also argued that it is unnecessary to use body-image distortion to explain the patient's dislike of her own body (Hsu & Sobkiewicz, in press-a), speculating (admittedly without much evidence) that perhaps certain central nervous system biochemical changes, which occur as a result of the self-imposed starvation, may intensify this fear of fatness, which occurs to a lesser extent in all dieters.

There is also no satisfactory explanation for the question of why some dieters develop restrictive anorexia nervosa while others develop bulimia nervosa. Perhaps the difference lies in their personality structure: There is some evidence to suggest that bulimics have greater difficulties with impulse control and affect regulation (see Chapter 2). If so, then the episodic binges may represent the periodic dyscontrol that bulimics experience when they attempt to go on a strict diet. Only a prospective study can settle this issue.

In summary, I have described the vicissitudes in the historical development of the concept of the eating disorders and their delineation from other psychiatric and physical conditions and from each other. It is upon the premise that the eating disorders are distinct entities that this book is written. I believe that studying the disorders as distinct entities is the approach most likely to yield further progress in the understanding and treatment of them.

2

Clinical Features

The onset of the eating disorders usually occurs in the late teens, and the female to male ratio is at least 10:1. The disorders almost always begin with dieting. For the anorectic, secondary amenorrhea may develop before there is any remarkable weight loss, although more commonly (perhaps for some 80% of patients) it coincides with or occurs shortly after a more determined effort to lose weight. Primary amenorrhea occurs if the onset of illness preceded menarche. In bulimia nervosa, amenorrhea develops in about one-third of the patients, while irregular menses occurs in another one-third. About 25% of anorectics and 40% of bulimics are actually overweight before the onset of the illness. It is clear, therefore, that the majority of patients are at a healthy weight when dieting begins, or at most are only a few pounds over their matched-population mean weight. After some initial weight loss and the attendant praise, admiration, and envy, the subsequent developments of the two disorders diverge. For the anorectic, the pursuit of thinness continues despite the escalating weight loss, and the fear of fatness actually increases, such that if she stays at the same weight from one day to the next she fears she will ultimately and inevitably become immensely obese. Usually she is quite uncertain about why she is so persistent with this willful dieting, except that she still feels too fat despite the weight loss or that she wants simply to keep increasing the safety margin between her actual weight and her ideal weight. Continued weight loss is considered a triumph, and staying at the same weight from one day to the next or gaining any weight generates despair and panic. The patient may look dejected or may actually complain of feeling depressed. Irritability, insomnia, social withdrawal, and preoccupation with food, dieting, and cooking increase as weight loss progresses. Most anorectics exercise feverishly to burn off calories, and the restlessness may continue until weight loss is severe. Crisp, Hsu, Harding, and Hartshorn (1980) found that within 2 years of the onset of restrictive anorexia nervosa some 40% of patients will develop bulimia, which then becomes a source of great distress to the patient and may precipitate attempted or actual suicide. The anorectic may counter the inevitable weight gain from the binges by purging, which, if her weight is still considerably below normal, may lead to cardiac arrest and death.

The bulimic patient may enter the bulimic cycle (see Figure 2.1) of fasting, bingeing, and purging by one of two ways. The majority, over 80%, develop the cycle by first giving in to the increasing urge to eat and thereafter self-inducing vomiting either because the fullness is intolerable or because they want to get rid of the calories. A smaller proportion actually begin vomiting to accelerate their weight loss, with the binges only coming later. In either case, the patient at first thinks she has hit upon the ideal solution to her dilemma: She can eat what she wants and still remain slim. Unfortunately, in time the binge-eating also becomes a response to stress and a way of coping with dysphoric feelings, such as anger, boredom, anxiety, depression, or being rejected. It may also be used to express impulsivity or rebelliousness. Some patients binge-eat when they are happy or excited. Most patients do not enjoy the vomiting or purging, although perhaps 10% feel that they serve to cleanse them of their guilt or relieve them of their tension. About two-thirds of bulimics regularly use vomiting to control their weight, while one-third predominantly abuse laxatives. Many, of course, combine both methods. The relative effectiveness of these weight-control measures obviously depends on many variables, but by and large laxative abuse is less effective and perhaps more likely to cause hypokalemia. Many bulimics also abuse diuretics, which, of course, do not get rid of any calories and are even more likely to cause an electrolyte disturbance. All purging may lead to rebound fluid retention, which perpetuates the fear of weight gain.

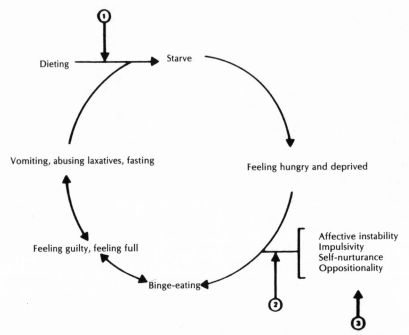

FIGURE 2.1.   The bulimic cycle (modified from Hsu & Holder, 1986). *Key to behavioral interventions:* (1) Diet and weight management, (2) strategies to tackle urges to binge, (3) social-skills training and interpersonal problem solving.

Some 40% of bulimics also abuse diet pills, alcohol, and/or street drugs.

It is unclear why only a small proportion of all dieters develop an eating disorder and, in the case of the anorectic, why the fear of fatness increases despite continuing weight loss. It is also unclear why some develop anorexia nervosa while others develop bulimia nervosa. Attempts to explain these issues by searching for personality and family variables are only beginning (see Chapter 4). The two disorders can occur in the same patient, or she may revert from one disorder to the other. Perhaps half of all anorectics binge and purge at least occasionally, but it is unclear how many would qualify for the *DSM-III-R* criterion of having at least two episodes a week. About 50% of normal-weight bulimics have a past history of anorexia nervosa (Hsu & Holder, 1986; Lacey, 1983; Russell, 1979), but clinical experience and follow-up data suggest that it is relatively rare for a normal-weight bulimic to revert to a pattern of restrictive anorexia nervosa (Hsu, 1988).

At this point it is important to review the Minnesota Experiment (Franklin, Schiele, Brozek, & Keys, 1948; Keys, Brozek, Henschel, Michelson, & Taylor, 1950; Schiele & Brozek, 1948) conducted more than 40 years ago. Thirty-six male conscientious objectors were selected from more than 100 volunteers to participate in a semistarvation experiment. These young men (mean age, 25.5 years) were in good health and at normal weight (average height, about 5′10″; average weight, about 175 pounds). During a 12-week adaptation period, they were allowed to eat what they wanted (on average, about 3,400 calories per day). Over the next 24 weeks of the study proper, they were given two meals a day (at 10:00 A.M. and 5:00 P.M.), totaling about 1,500 calories according to a 3-day rotating menu in order to simulate the meal conditions of a European concentration camp. After a few weeks, all the men became preoccupied with food and eating, many also developing an avid interest in recipes and cooking. Increased consumption of coffee, tea, chewing gum, tobacco, and table salt occurred, and some developed bizarre eating habits and unusual food combinations. Many reported that they were caught between wanting to gulp their food to satisfy their hunger and wanting to prolong the pleasure of eating for as long as possible. Some dreamed about eating and food (including one who dreamed of cannibalism). All reported increased lethargy, poor concentration, loss of sexual interest, increased irritability, moodiness, and insomnia. Four became very depressed, and one developed what appeared to be a bipolar disorder; the latter and another subject had to be hospitalized. A third was hospitalized after making two attempts at self-mutilation, during one of which he cut three fingers off his left hand with an ax. Several admitted to breaking their diet and bingeing outside of the experimental situation, and at least one binged on food taken from garbage cans and vomited. In order to prevent the breaking of the diet, a buddy system was then instituted, although this caused some resentment among the men. At the end of the 24 weeks they were then continued on a rehabilitation program, with a third of the subjects eating about 2,000 calories daily; another third, 2,500; and the final third, 3,000. After 6 weeks it was obvious that the men were not improving in terms of their mood and energy, and more calories were added; but despite this, the men did not recover completely by the end of the 12-week rehabilitation period. Preoccupation with food, messing with food, and poor table manners, such as licking of plates, persisted. Twelve men then volunteered to go on another 6 weeks of rehabilitation. Over the weekends of this second rehabilitation period they were allowed to eat whatever they wanted, and the men ate practically continuously, consuming up to 10,000 calories per day. They ate until they were physically too full but somehow still did not feel satiated. Some of the men also became concerned about fat accumulation in their abdomens and buttocks. All the men were followed up a year later, by which time they had recovered from their bizarre eating habits and moodiness. This experiment demonstrated dramatically the effects of prolonged semistarvation on mood and behavior in normal subjects. It is clear that the symptoms of anorexia nervosa and bulimia nervosa, except for the weight phobia and the restless hyperactivity, are directly caused by the self-imposed starvation. Treatment of these conditions must therefore necessarily include nutritional replenishment.

EXPERIENTIAL ASPECTS

Numerous authors have commented on the difficulty that anorectics have in discussing their feelings and thoughts. In attempting to make sense of this curious experience, many authors have combined the patients' statements with their own interpretations. In fact, apart from anecdotal descriptions, there is actually very little objective data on the anorectic experience. Denial of illness is almost universal: The anorectic will insist that she is eating enough and that she looks just fine, if not too fat. Even when emaciated, an anorectic may point to her abdomen or her thighs, claiming that there is still too much fat. Such denial is most common among adolescent patients who have not had a long duration of illness. The fact that she is suffering from the effects of starvation is betrayed, however, by her interest in cooking and food, the consumption of large quantities of low-calorie liquids, and the chewing of gum. Sometimes she will admit that she thinks about food, perhaps even dreams about it, but such preoccupation is always countered by other activities, such as exercising or schoolwork. Some anorectics may admit to a feeling of emptiness, worthlessness, helplessness, or hopelessness. Others, however, seem to lack the language for talking about such feelings and experiences (Levenkron, 1983). What the anorectic may be more willing to talk about is her fear of fatness, her despair and panic if she gains weight, and her exhilaration and sense of triumph when she has lost more weight. Some anorectics, usually older women who have had some psychotherapy, will identify their dieting as competence and control, claiming that their weight and eating habits are a small part of their lives that they can successfully control. Some admit to feeling special, different, or unique because of their thinness. Some enjoy the attention, concern, and envy they receive. A few may even acknowledge that such dieting demonstrates to themselves and to others their autonomy: No one can make them eat or gain weight. Most anorectics, however, at least in the early stages of the illness, cannot explain their fear of fatness; they can only emphatically restate it.

Upon recovery, two anorectics shared the following reasons for their dieting. At a follow-up interview a 26-year-old patient said she started dieting at age 16 because of her acute embarrassment over the difference in the size of her breasts. She dieted in the hope of making them look more equal. She was never able to discuss this fear in her 2 years of inpatient and outpatient therapy, although she did make a substantial recovery during that period. The focus of the individual and family therapy was on the death of the mother prior to the patient's onset of illness and a presumed sexual relationship between the patient and her father. She had finally undergone breast reconstructive surgery 2 years before the follow-up.

A 24-year-old married ex-patient said during a follow-up interview that the onset of her dieting at age 16 was related to homosexual advances made toward her by a classmate in her boarding school. She could not, however, explain how the severe dieting could have helped her in dealing with that situation. She never discussed this issue with her therapist in 4 months of intensive inpatient therapy, which focused, in addition to weight restoration, on the mother's promiscuity.

Researchers may, of course, say that such retrospective, anecdotal reports are of questionable value in our understanding of the illness. The fact remains, however, that there are very few objective data on the phenomenological experience of the anorectic during her illness.

In contrast, somewhat more is known about the phenomenon of bulimia nervosa from an experiential perspective (Abraham & Beumont, 1982a; Hsu, in press; Mitchell & Laine, 1985). The precipitants of a particular binge, based on the recollection of bulimic patients, can generally be divided into: (1) certain dysphoric states (i.e., emotional); (2) certain situations or the anticipation of being in such situations (i.e., social or situational); and (3) feelings related to food and hunger (i.e., physiological). The most common dysphoric moods that trigger a binge are tension or anxiety; other identified feelings include being unhappy (depressed), being bored and lonely, feeling empty, being frustrated, feeling rejected, and being angry. The tension before a binge may be induced by the environment or may be related to the effort to suppress the urge to binge. Being alone is the situation most likely to precipitate a binge, while the next most common is being with the family, particularly the mother. Being surrounded with plenty of food also commonly precipitates a binge. Patients most frequently binge in the evening or afternoon when they are alone and feel bored and tired; very often they are also starved from having dieted all day. Only 10% of bulimics eat more than one meal a day. Finally, binges are often triggered because patients crave certain foods, especially those they have been depriving themselves of.

Once the urge to binge is triggered, the patient will do almost anything to have a binge. She may try to get rid of the people around her so she can binge alone. Most commonly she binges in her own home, usually in the kitchen or while watching television. If there is no food available in the home, she may visit several grocery or convenience stores so that no one will notice that she has purchased such vast quantities of food. Alternatively, a binge may follow upon what was intended to be a normal meal. Once the first bite is taken, the most common thought is, "Now that I have blown my diet, I might as well make the most of the situation and go all the way." Some may express bewilderment over their loss of control: "Why am I doing this?" Guilt and self-condemnation are common. Paradoxically, there is sometimes a sense of relief, even of liberation or triumph: "I can eat what I want to and no one can stop me." Some describe the food as giving them a feeling of nurturance. Perhaps one out of four continues to binge so that she can vomit: "The fuller I feel the easier it is to purge." Others describe a sense of oblivion, of being able to forget about problems. However, within about half-an-hour, negative feelings of guilt and disgust take over; the patient then feels uncomfortably full and will resort to vomiting or taking laxatives.

Only a minority of patients actually enjoy the purge. Most, perhaps 80%, describe it as necessary for getting rid of calories (i.e., to relieve them of the anxiety regarding weight gain). The rest may feel that the purging itself can relieve them of tension, guilt, and dysphoria. They may describe the tiredness after the purge as relaxing. Most patients then regain a new sense of resolve to start over again, although some may go on to another binge-and-purge episode. About one-third fall asleep after an episode.

The *DSM-III-R* criteria for bulimia nervosa specify a minimum frequency of two episodes of bingeing per week, with an accompaniment of vomiting, laxative abuse, and/or severe dieting. Occasional binge-eating as defined in the *DSM-III-R* is probably quite common among young women and men (Halmi, Falk, & Schwartz, 1981; Pyle et al., 1983), but it remains unclear whether such behavior will later evolve into bulimia nervosa. Among patients who meet criteria for bulimia nervosa, most are bingeing and purging once a day, although a few may have up to ten or more episodes per day. The frequency of episodes may fluctuate, and binge-free periods lasting a few weeks to a few months are not uncommon.

Recently, direct objective study of bulimic behavior in laboratory settings has been attempted by several groups (e.g., Kaye, Gwirtsman, George, Weiss, & Jimerson, 1986; Mitchell & Laine, 1985; Rosen, Leitenberg, Fisher, & Khazam, 1986; Walsh, Kissileff, Cassidy, & Dantzic, 1989). By and large, these studies have confirmed that when asked to eat as much as they could, bulimic patients ate significantly more than normal controls (a binge commonly varied between a few thousand to 20,000 calories). Although patients and controls had similar intake when asked to eat normally, bulimic patients felt significantly more hungry after these normal meals than controls. Somewhat surprisingly, the macronutrient content of a binge meal is similar to that of a non-binge meal: 50% carbohydrate, 40% fat, 10% protein. Thus, in a laboratory setting, the difference between a binge and a normal meal lies primarily in the amount of food consumed, not in the nutritional content. These laboratory studies may be used to objectively evaluate the effects of treatment.

ONSET OF ILLNESS

Clinical experience and epidemiological studies both suggest that the mean age of onset of anorexia nervosa is about 17 years, although it may begin before the age of 10 or after the age of 40. However, the onset of illness is an event that is hard to define in anorexia nervosa. Most published series take the onset of severe dieting or significant weight loss to be the onset of illness, while some others include also the onset of amenorrhea. For most patients, severe and determined dieting is preceded by about 6 months of sporadic dieting and followed a few months later by the onset of amenorrhea (Crisp, Hsu, Harding, & Hartshorn, 1980). However, simply determining the mean age of onset may obscure individual patterns of onset. In their series of 105 patients, Halmi, Casper, Eckert, Goldberg, and Davis (1979) found a bimodal distribution, with peaks of onset at 14 and 18 years. These investigators speculate that it is at these ages that dependency on the family is most greatly challenged. Around age 14 the patients are entering a high school system that is, by comparison, large, impersonal, and demanding. At age 18 the patients are expected to become even more independent. The authors further speculate that the desire to be thin is heightened at such times of uncertainty. A younger age of onset is associated with less weight loss, more bizarre food habits and obsessions about food and cooking, and greater overestimation of body width. These features may, however, simply be a function of age. For instance, overestimation of body width is a characteristic even of nonanorectic young girls, who are simply less accurate than older girls in their estimation of body width (Bentovim, Whitehead, & Crisp, 1979). Most anorectic patients have had a duration of illness of about 4 years by the time they seek treatment. Several reports of the onset of illness in older women have been published (see Hsu & Zimmer, 1988).

For bulimia nervosa the mean age of onset is around 18 years, although, again, it may begin before the age of 10 or after the age of 40. There is some indication that onset later than age 25 may be associated with more chemical dependency problems, suicidal attempts, and depressive symptoms (Mitchell, Hatsukami, Pyle, Eckert, & Soll, 1987). Thus even within the syndrome of bulimia nervosa there may be some distinct subgroups. In general, the bulimia is preceded by a variable period of dieting and followed by the onset of purging to counter the weight gain. However, no study has been published that specifically examines the age of onset of each event. Duration of illness for patients who seek treatment is again about 4 years.

PRECIPITATING EVENTS

Bruch (1973) found that most of her patients could recall the event that made them feel too fat and convinced them of the urgent need to lose weight. In most of the published series, significant life events that seem to lead to the development of anorexia nervosa occur in from one-third (Beck & Brochner-Mortensen, 1954) to two-thirds of cases (Kay & Leigh, 1954; Morgan & Russell, 1975). In general, they are related to being teased for being fat, sexual and other interpersonal conflicts, separation from family, personal illness or failure, and family difficulties (Crisp, Hsu, Harding, & Hartshorn, 1980; Dally, 1969; Kay & Leigh, 1954; Morgan & Russell, 1975; Theander, 1970). Of the family difficulties, Kalucy, Crisp, and Harding (1977) found that death, illness, or marital problems commonly precede the onset of illness, as do the occurrence of acting-out behavior, sexual or otherwise, by a parent or sibling. Early or recent sexual trauma has been postulated as a significant precipitating event, but its occurrence is apparently no more frequent among individuals with eating disorders than among those in therapy for other reasons (Finn, Hartman, Leon, & Larson, 1986).

Both collection and analysis of retrospective data on precipitating events are fraught with difficulties. In the absence of a standardized interview, the findings are likely to be biased by the investigator's perspective. For instance, onset of menarche is identified as a stressful event by Crisp, Hsu, Harding, and Hartshorn (1980) in 40% of the patients, but it is not mentioned by any of the other investigators. Underreporting and overreporting are other problems that lead to biased results. Absence of a proper control group affects most of the studies reviewed. In a more carefully controlled study, Strober (1984) found that stressful life events in an 18-month period prior to the onset of illness was significantly more common in a group of 25 teenage bulimic anorectics than in a matched control group of 25 teenage restrictive anorectics. The most common stressors identified by interview were change in acceptance by peers, arguments between parents, arguments with parents, serious parental illness, serious personal illness, not having extracurricular activities, father's absence from home, and being involved with drugs. In view of the young age of the cohort, menarche is also likely to be a significant event, but Strober does not mention it.

In my view, the onset of an eating disorder is unlikely to be related to a specific stress or event, although the patient almost always responds to such a stressful event by dieting (see Chapter 4). However, since stressful life events are generally more common before the onset of a psychiatric disorder, we can expect the same to hold true for an eating disorder. It seems that most of the stressful events that precipitate an eating disorder are related to the life events of an adolescent.

MENSTRUAL DISTURBANCES

By *DSM-III-R* definition, all anorectics have at least 3 months of amenorrhea during the course of their illness, and, as already mentioned, this has been the traditional view as well. In most patients weight loss occurs before the onset of amenorrhea; sometimes the two events are concurrent; and in a small proportion of patients, perhaps 10% to 20% (Kay & Leigh, 1954; Theander, 1970), amenorrhea actually occurs before the onset of any weight loss. While such findings may appear puzzling, one has to recognize the inherent difficulties involved in gathering reliable dietary data retrospectively from anorectic patients, who tend to deny their difficulties (Beumont, Abraham, & Simson, 1981). In any event, whether amenorrhea occurs before or after the onset of illness has no bearing on the course and outcome of the disorder. In bulimia nervosa, menstrual disturbances are common, with amenorrhea occurring in perhaps 25% to 50% of patients and irregular menses in another 25% to 50% (Fairburn & Cooper, 1984; Garner, Garfinkel, & O'Shaughnessy, 1985; Johnson, Stuckey, Lewis, & Schwartz, 1982; Lacey, 1983; Pirke, Schweiger, Laessle, Fichter, & Wolfram, 1987; Weiss & Ebert, 1983). The exact proportion of patients reporting amenorrhea and oligomenorrhea varies between series, of course, and depends on such factors as patient selection and actual body weight at the time of the study. Apparently a past history of anorexia nervosa is not associated with menstrual irregularity in a normal-weight bulimic patient.

The pathogenesis of amenorrhea in anorexia nervosa has long been a subject of debate. Amenorrhea occurs in response to nonspecific emotional stress, malnutrition, and weight loss. Two to five percent of college-age women report having amenorrhea and 10% or so oligomenorrhea (Bachman & Kemmann, 1982). It is unclear whether the menstrual irregularities are associated with dietary restriction or emotional stress. For women confined to concentration camps during the Second World War, amenorrhea occurred initially in about 60% (Sydenham, 1946); although this was apparently not associated with weight loss, it was associated with changing to a diet of decreased protein and increased carbohydrate intake. Thus emotional shock may be assumed to have been primarily responsible for the amenorrhea. This initial amenorrhea cleared up in the majority of women within 6 months. A second wave of amenorrhea occurred when there was a subsequent decrease in both caloric and protein intake. Unfortunately, neither the number of women who developed this second wave of amenorrhea nor their body weights were reported. In women refugees who suffered starvation, amenorrhea was universal (Grieve, 1946). Unfortunately, however, details regarding body weight were again not reported, although it can be assumed that weight loss occurred in the majority of such individuals. Recent studies (Pirke et al., 1987) have shown that even a mild weight loss of two kilograms in a healthy woman may result in disturbed hormonal secretion and impaired follicular development. Amenorrhea can be expected to develop in 80% of women who have lost 12% of their ideal weight (average, about 8 kilogram) (Pirke et al., 1987).

In a study of 36 women with anorexia nervosa and 37 with normal-weight bulimia nervosa, Treasure (1988), using pelvic ultrasound scans, found amenorrhea to be associated with a cystic appearance of the ovaries, which represents a regression of the ovarian structure to a prepubertal state. Adequate weight gain causes the reappearance of a dominant follicle during the menstrual cycle and return of menstruation. This study demonstrates clearly that the amenorrhea in anorexia and bulimia nervosa is related at least in part to regressive changes in the ovaries (most probably secondary to persistent hypothalamic dysfunction) and that recovery of the ovaries occurs with weight gain and therefore takes time. Nevertheless, some investigators still believe that the amenorrhea in anorexia nervosa (and bulimia nervosa) may represent a primary hypothalamic dysfunction not entirely related to the state of malnutrition because it frequently precedes any obvious weight loss and it may persist despite apparent weight recovery (e.g., Russell, 1977a). Before concluding that these findings indicate the presence of a primary hypothalamic disorder, clinicians need to bear in mind the following issues:

1. As already mentioned, it is notoriously difficult to gather retrospective data from anorectic patients, particularly a reliable dietary history (Crisp & Stonehill, 1971). This was well illustrated by the study of Beumont and colleagues (1981). Two patients in their series initially indicated that amenorrhea had occurred before weight loss, but subsequent careful history taking found that months of chaotic eating had preceded the amenorrhea. Minor weight fluctuations, which have been found by recent studies to be associated with abnormal hormonal secretion and follicular development, may therefore not be reported by the patient.

2. Despite apparent weight recovery, many anorectics continue to binge, vomit, and starve. Such eating disturbances most probably prevent a full recovery of the hypothalamic–pituitary–ovarian axis function (Katz, Boyar, Roffwarg, Hellman, & Weiner, 1978; Treasure, 1988). Furthermore, restoration to premorbid or matched-population mean weight rather than ideal weight may be necessary for menstruation to resume (Crisp & Stonehill, 1971). A modest amount of weight gain (mean, 3.6 kg) is associated with onset of ovalatory menstrual cycles in women presenting with amenorrhea to a gynecological clinic (Knuth, Hull, & Jacobs, 1977). Conversely, as we have already mentioned, a modest amount of weight loss is associated with menstrual irregularity (Pirke, Schweiger, & Fichter, 1987). Thus, persistent amenorrhea may occur in those who are apparently weight-recovered but who are still bingeing and purging, or if they are still below their optimal weight.

3. There is some evidence to suggest that the recovery of hypothalamic function may occur in sequence and full recovery may take time (Wakeling, DeSouza, & Beardwood, 1977). However, in the study by Wakeling and colleagues (1977) only three out of seven patients who maintained their weight over a 6-month period menstruated (and it is unclear whether the patients were at or above their matched-population mean weight and whether they had a balanced and regular dietary intake).

In sum, although it remains possible that the primary hypothalamic disorder may exist in anorexia nervosa and bulimia nervosa, the evidence for this is not strong.

BODY WEIGHT IN ANOREXIA NERVOSA AND BULIMIA NERVOSA

The *DSM-III-R* does not specify how low the weight has to be to qualify for the diagnosis of anorexia nervosa, and it has eliminated weight as a criterion for bulimia nervosa. In most series of anorectics the patient's body weight at presentation is below 85% of matched-population mean weight, with a mean of 70% to 75%. The lowest weight during an anorectic illness is usually 65% to 70% of matched-population mean weight. For bulimics, the majority (about 70%) are within 10% of matched-population mean weight, with the remaining 30% approximately equally divided between being 10% to 25% underweight and 10% to 25% overweight (Fairburn & Cooper, 1984; Johnson et al., 1982; Mitchell, Hatsukami, Eckert, & Pyle, 1985). The question of whether bulimia nervosa in an underweight individual should be classified as anorexia nervosa will be discussed in Chapter 5.

DEVELOPMENTAL HISTORY, PERSONALITY, AND SEXUALITY

Retrospective data are notoriously difficult to collect reliably, and researchers use different criteria for interpreting their findings. Furthermore, the parameters used in such studies are crude and thus unlikely to yield data on more subtle disturbances. Not surprisingly, therefore, the findings on developmental history are often conflicting and their significance, unclear.

The data on the birthweight of anorectics are confusing; both low and high birthweights have been reported (Crisp, 1965; Wall, 1959). Mild childhood and adolescent obesity are probably more common than excessive thinness, a point on which the major series are in agreement. The data on childhood feeding difficulties are also conflicting, but the majority of patients probably do not have any eating difficulties. For bulimics, most studies find a significant proportion to be premorbidly overweight (Beumont et al., 1976; Garfinkel et al., 1980). A few studies have found that bulimics require less calories to maintain their weight than restrictive anorectics (Kaye et al., 1986; Stordy, Marks, Kalucy, & Crisp, 1977), a finding that, if confirmed, may explain the bulimics' tendency to become overweight.

Most anorectics are described as perfect children, a situation taken by some to reflect major developmental deficits in the development of the self and a symbiotic relationship with an overinvolved significant other. Unfortunately, such reports are retrospective and anecdotal. Clinical impressions suggest that these patients are often compliant and perfectionistic, but usually socially and interpersonally inept. Bruch (1973) and others (e.g., Crisp, 1980; Palazzoli, 1978) have described their pervasive sense of ineffectiveness, uncertainty about their internal sensations and feelings, and lack of autonomy. Their obsessiveness and emotional overcontrol are deemed to be attempts on their part to control their core deficiencies. In contrast, bulimics may have more impulse control problems even before the onset of the illness (Mitchell, Hatsukami, Eckert, & Pyle, 1985).

Objective studies to identify the personality characteristics of eating-disorder patients are few in number. A major consideration is the contamination of personality measures by the psychopathology of the illness. For instance, recovery from anorexia nervosa is associated with a decrease in neuroticism and introversion (Crisp, Hsu, & Stonehill, 1979), features that have been considered characteristic of the personality of anorectic patients (Smart, Beumont, & George, 1976). In an attempt to overcome this problem, Strober (1981) studied 50 adolescent anorectics with a recent onset of illness and used matched groups of depressed and antisocial adolescent females as comparisons. Responses on the Cattell High School Personality Questionnaire (Cattell & Cattell, 1969) indicated that anorectics are characterized by greater conformity, neurotic anxieties, control of emotionality, and stimulus avoidance. In an earlier study comparing 8 adolescent vomiters with 14 abstainers, also with a recent onset of illness, Strober (1980) found that, on a variety of personality and psychopathology measures, the two anorectic groups were more obsessive, had a higher need for social approval, and were less psychological-minded and flexible when compared to depressed and personality-disordered adolescent patients. However, they also showed a higher sense of responsibility, self-control, conformance, and intellectual efficiency. Compared to the restrictors, the vomiting subgroup exhibited greater impairment in self-control, greater sociability, and greater adaptability and flexibilty in their thinking and social behavior. These findings are thus by and large consistent with clinical impression and with findings in older patients (e.g., Garner, Garfinkel, & O'Shaughnessy, 1985).

For bulimia nervosa, most of the studies have used the Minnesota Multiphasic Personality Inventory, which is arguably more a measure of symptomatology than personality. Furthermore, because the studies were conducted in older patients with a longer duration of illness, "contamination" is more likely. Reviewing the findings from several studies, Johnson and Connors (1987, p. 75) suggest that the bulimic anorectic is the most disturbed. The normal-weight bulimics, although showing less overall psychopathology, are similar to the bulimic anorectics in terms of their vulnerability to impulsivity. In contrast, restricting anorectics have a greater tendency to be depressed, to avoid close interpersonal relationships, and to fear the loss of impulse control. In summary, the objective personality measures of bulimics are again consistent with clinical impression. Whether these tendencies reflect premorbid personality and whether they persist after recovery remain to be studied.

Practically all the investigators have suggested that, as a group, anorectics are sexually inactive and uninterested in sex. Some investigators have found that bulimic anorectics are more sexually active than restrictive anorectics (Abraham & Beumont, 1982b; Garfinkel et al., 1980; Russell, 1979), but the two groups seem equally negative in their attitude toward sex (Leon, Lucas, Colligan, Ferndinande, & Kamp, 1985). Normal-weight bulimics are similar to age-matched controls in most aspects of sexual attitude and behavior (Abraham et al., 1985; Johnson & Connors, 1987): However, the onset of bulimia seems to be associated with the loss of sexual interest for some and an increase for others (Johnson & Connors, 1987; Mitchell, Hatsukami, Pyle, & Eckert, 1986).

The issue of sexuality is of particular interest to investigators for several reasons. Some speculate that the fear of sexuality is sometimes the primary reason for the development of the avoidant response of anorexia nervosa (e.g., Crisp, 1980; Sours, 1980). Others consider it to be related to the wider issue of adolescent identity, which is problematic for the would-be anorectic (Bruch, 1973; Palazzoli, 1978). However, many factors may influence the development of sexual attitudes and behavior; those that are relevant to the eating disorders include state of nutrition and weight, age of onset of illness, age of menarche, self-perception, presence of depression, personality characteristics, and family and social background. For instance, with the development of bulimia nervosa some patients may become less interested in sex because of concurrent major depression, while others may become more interested because they feel more attractive as a result of their weight loss. Obviously the topic needs to be studied further.

OTHER PSYCHIATRIC DIAGNOSES

For the restrictive anorectic, food-related obsessive–compulsive features, such as constant preoccupation with food and ritualistic food preparation, are common and are probably due to the effects of starvation. Such thoughts and actions are, however, not usually experienced as intrusive or senseless and thus are not typical of obsessive–compulsive features. Nonfood-related obsessive–compulsive features, such as repeated hand washing and checking if the door is locked, may also occur. It is unclear, however, what proportion of the patients would qualify for an actual obsessive–compulsive disorder. Social anxiety, usually expressed as due to embarrassment over fatness, is also common, particularly among bulimics. Again, it is unclear what proportion would qualify for an anxiety disorder. The issue of depression in the eating disorders has already been discussed in the previous chapter. In our experience, about 20% of anorectics and 40% of bulimics meet criteria for major depression. A somewhat higher than expected proportion of eating-disorder patients, perhaps about 5% overall, develop a psychotic illness with schizophrenic and affective features that run independently of the anorectic illness. Alcohol and substance abuse, as well as such other conduct problems as stealing, occur in perhaps a third of all bulimic patients. Finally, clinical reports suggest that many bulimics may qualify for a diagnosis of borderline personality disorder, manifesting such behaviors as mood lability, impulsivity, explosive interpersonal relationships, and self-mutilation (e.g., Levin & Hyler, 1986). However, Pope, Frankenburg, Hudson, Jonas, and Yurgelun-Todd (1987), in a controlled study, found that a secondary diagnosis of borderline personality disorder occurred only in 1.9% of female bulimic patients according to strict criteria, compared to 4.5% in a control group of depressed female outpatients. Our own experience suggests that about 15% of normal-weight bulimics qualify for a diagnosis of borderline personality disorder.

THE ISSUE OF BODY-IMAGE DISTURBANCE IN ANOREXIA AND BULIMIA NERVOSA

The *DSM-III* listed the disturbance of body image as the third of five necessary criteria for anorexia nervosa. This has been changed to "disturbance in the way in which one's body weight, size or shape is experienced" in the *DSM-III-R* (APA, 1987, p. 67). The idea that there is a disturbance of body image in anorexia nervosa was first described by Bruch (1962) in an intuitive attempt to explain the intriguing pursuit of thinness in these patients. However, her definition of body-image disturbance is broad and includes disturbances in a wide range of perceptions and affects: awareness of the bodily self, interoceptive awareness of bodily sensations, control over bodily functions, affective reaction to the reality of bodily configuration, and self-rating of the desirability of one's body by others (Bruch, 1973). This concept has generated much research in two major areas: perception of body dimensions and attitudes and affect toward one's body. Although almost never explicitly stated, the purpose of these studies is to investigate if the patient's claim of feeling fat, despite her normal or emaciated size may be related to either: (1) a perceptual overestimation of her actual body size, or (2) a disparaging attitude toward her body.

Studies in body-dimension perceptions have mainly used four techniques: image marking, analogue methods, optical distortion, and kinesthetic measures. Studies in bodily attitudes and affect have utilized a variety of self-rating measures and questionnaires. Unfortunately, none of the studies reviewed specifically addressed what body image is, or whether the parameters studied are in fact measures of body image. Reviewing the findings of 19 studies published between 1983 and 1988, Hsu and Sobkiewicz (in press-a) found that for anorectics, seven studies found no difference between patients and controls, two found greater variability in the patients' estimates of bodily dimensions, and five found greater overestimation in the patients. For bulimics, five found no difference, one found greater variability, and nine found greater overestimation on the part of the bulimics. Further, the review found overestimation of body dimensions to be influenced by a multitude of factors unrelated to an eating disorder: sex and age of subject, mood and self-esteem, masculinity and femininity, whether the individuals based estimates on what they thought or how they felt, the methods used for studying body-size estimation, and a host of other factors. For the attitudinal/affect studies, the findings were unanimous in indicating that the patients (whether anorectic or bulimic) were more negative than controls toward their bodies.

The authors concluded that (1) overestimation of bodily dimensions is not pathognomonic of either anorexia or bulimia nervosa; (2) overestimation of body dimensions is influenced by a multitude of factors independent of eating-disorder symptomatology; (3) overestimation of body dimensions, even if present, may not explain the patient's fear of fatness since the latter is often idiosyncratic (e.g., a patient feels fat because the inner parts of her thighs touch each other when she sits) and occurs even in those who estimated their body dimensions accurately; (4) there is no evidence that overestimation of body size, even if present, occurs because of a disturbance in body image; (5) although body disparagement is very common among eating-disorder patients, it is unnecessary to explain it by the ill-defined concept of body-image disturbance, that is, there is no evidence that patients dislike their bodies because of such a disturbance; and (6) it is unclear how body disparagement and fear of fatness are related since the two may occur independently of each other, particularly among anorectics. However, it is conceivable that feelings of fatness could be an expression of body disparagement. The authors suggest that, in order to avoid further confusion, the fear of fatness and negative attitudes and affects toward the body should simply be described as such without reference to body image.

FAMILY CHARACTERISTICS

The eating disorders run in families. Theander (1970) reported that 6.6% of the siblings of a series of 94 female anorectic patients had the disorder, while Crisp, Hsu, Harding, and Hartshorn (1980) found 14%

of the mothers and 9% of the fathers of female anorectics to have probable anorexia nervosa. Hudson, Pope, Jonas, and Yurgelun-Todd (1983), in a study of 14 anorectic probands, found 5.9% of the first-degree relatives to have an eating disorder (either anorexia nervosa, bulimia, or atypical eating disorder), while the familial prevalence of eating disorders in bulimics ($n = 55$) and anorectic bulimic patients ($n = 20$) were 4.8% and 6.1%, respectively. However, the authors did not report the prevalence rate for relatives of controls. Gershon and colleagues (1984), in a study of 24 anorectics and 43 normals, found the age-corrected rate of anorexia nervosa to be about 4% and bulimia to be about 8% among the patients' relatives; the rate among control-group relatives was about 1% (e.g., one relative had bulimia). In a carefully conducted study, Strober, Morrell, Burroughs, Salkin, and Jacobs (1985) interviewed the first- and second-degree relatives of 60 anorectics (39 restrictive and 21 bulimic) and 95 psychiatric controls (45 with an affective disorder, 22 with schizophrenia, 28 with a conduct disorder). All together, 27% of the anorectic families and 6% of the control families had at least one relative with an eating disorder; the figures for anorexia nervosa were 22% and 3% and for bulimia nervosa 12% and 4%, respectively. Ninety-seven percent of the affected relatives of both anorectics and controls were female. Expressed differently, female relatives of anorectics have a fivefold greater risk for developing an eating disorder compared to those of the psychiatric non-anorectic controls (9.7% vs. 1.9%). There was no significant increase in risk among the male relatives of the anorectics. Thus, if we take the prevalence in the general population of anorexia nervosa to be about 1% and bulimia nervosa to be about 2%, then the first- and second-degree relatives of eating-disorder patients are perhaps four to five times more likely than the general public to develop an eating disorder themselves. Dividing the anorectic probands into restrictor and bulimic subgroups, Strober (1985) and his colleagues found a somewhat higher prevalence of familial eating disorders among the bulimics than among the restrictors (13% vs. 8%). They also found that severe restrictive anorexia nervosa was confined to relatives of the restrictive probands, while bulimia was much more common in relatives of bulimic probands. The authors speculate that the transmission of bulimia may be quite specific within certain bulimic anorectic families.

However, the most common psychiatric illness among the relatives of eating-disorder patients is an affective disorder (see Table 2.1).

TABLE 2.1. Family History of Affective Disorders in Eating-Disorder Patients

	Patients				Patient relatives	Controls	Control relatives	Method	Findings
	AN	BN	Both						
Biederman et al. (1985) (Reanalysis of Rivinus data)	38	—	—		166 (1°)	23 Normals	81 (1°)	Nonblind interview	Significant increase in UP and substance abuse in *depressed* AN families only
Gershon et al. (1984)	24 (11 also bulimic)				99 (1°)	43 medically ill	265 (1°)	Case-controlled blind interview & FH	(1) Significant increase of UP, BP, and schizoaffective in AN families (2) Increase in UP in families not correlated with depression in AN patients, whereas BP and schizoaffective are (3) No difference in family prevalence for restrictors and bulimics

Study							Method	Findings
Hudson et al. (1983)	14	55	20	420 (1°)	33 BP, 39 Schiz, 15 BD	499 (1°)	Nonblind interview & FH	Significant increase of UP, BP, & ALc in AN families
Rivinis et al. (1984)	40	—	—	545 (1° & 2°)	23 Normals	217 (1° & 2°)	Nonblind interview	Significant increase of UP and substance abuse in AN families
Stern et al. (1984)	—	27	—	368 (1° & 2°)	27 normals	384 (1° & 2°)	Nonblind interview & FH	No increase of UP or BP or substance abuse in BN families
Winokur et al. (1980)	25	—	—	192 (1° & 2°)	25 normals	177 (1° & 2°)	Nonblind interview & FH	Significant increase of UP and BP in AN families

Note. AN = anorexia nervosa; BN = bulimia nervosa; UP = unipolar disorder; BP = bipolar disorder; ALc = alcoholism; BD = borderline personality disorder; FH = family history.

For the families of anorectic patients, the lifetime prevalence of unipolar depression is three times higher than for the general population (5% to 10% for relatives of normals, 15% to 25% for anorectic families). This is also true—it is contradicted only in one study by Stern and colleagues (1984)—for relatives of bulimic patients. The evidence for an increase in familial prevalence for bipolar disorder and alcohol and substance abuse disorders is also substantial (Table 2.1). Of the studies reviewed, only Rivinis and colleagues (1984) and Stern and colleagues (1984) found no increase in the familial prevalence of bipolar disorder, while Winokur, March, and Mendels (1980) and Stern and colleagues (1984) found no increase in alcohol or substance abuse. Earlier, Strober, Salkin, Burroughs, and Morrell (1982) had compared the first- and second-degree relatives of 35 bulimic anorectics and 35 restrictive anorectics and found familial alcohol and substance abuse to be significantly higher in the former group. It is, however, still unclear whether the various subgroups of eating-disorder patients show differential familial loadings for affective and substance abuse disorders. For instance, some investigators have found that the familial prevalence of affective disorders is higher among anorectics who are depressed (Biederman et al., 1985; Strober & Katz, 1988) and among bulimic anorectics (Strober et al., 1982), but other investigators were unable to confirm such findings (Gershon et al., 1984). These conflicting findings point either to a difference in the patient populations studied or, more likely, to the problematic reliability of collecting psychiatric data on family members.

Basically all the twin studies favor a genetic predisposition to the development of anorexia nervosa, although the exact mechanism of the predisposition is unknown. However, there is an intricate interplay between genetics and environment, and the role of the family both as the gene carrier and the environment for the genesis of the disorder deserves intensive investigation. (Data from twin studies are reviewed in Chapter 4.)

The idea that somehow the family environment is detrimental to the recovery of the patient was espoused by most if not all of the early writers. They therefore almost always recommended isolation of the patient from the family, and in the nineteenth century Charcot went to the extent of refusing to treat a patient unless she was hospitalized. By and large the more recent writings on the families of eating-disorder patients have centered on (1) the parents' own psychopathology, (2) the family interactive process, and (3) the "value" of the illness to the family.

Apart from the overt psychiatric disorders already described, most recent writings have emphasized the parents' more covert and buried psychopathology despite their apparent healthy adjustment. Bruch (1973), for instance, described the parents as controlling and experience-denying, often frustrated in their aspirations, and convinced of being only second-best. She also described them as using the child to cover up their sense of inadequacy, and as competing with each other about who was making greater sacrifices for the family. Palazzoli (1978), in accordance with Bruch's views, found the parents to conceal behind their facade of respectability and solidarity a deep sense of disillusion with themselves and each other and to overcompensate for such feelings, which they denied, by dedicating themselves to doing good, often in competition with each other. Crisp (1967, 1977) and his colleagues (Kalucy et al., 1977) found that the parents were confronting their own midlife crises just as the child was entering adolescence and therefore felt threatened by the rekindling of their long-buried but unresolved identity conflicts. Sexual difficulties were serious in some 40% of the parents. Along with other authors, such as Bruch (1973), Kay and Leigh (1954), Kalucy and colleagues (1977), and Nemiah (1950), he found a high prevalence of abnormal parental attitudes toward weight, diet, and shape. Apart from these clinical descriptions, controlled studies are unfortunately rare. Crisp, Harding, and McGuinness (1974), in a prospective study of 22 patients and their parents, found the parents to become significantly more anxious and depressed on the Middlesex Hospital Questionnaire as the patient was restored to a normal adolescent weight through intensive inpatient treatment. Poor outcome at 6 months was correlated with higher initial parental depression, maternal obsessiveness, and parental extroversion. Garfinkel, Garner, Rose, et al. (1983) compared the parents of 23 anorectics with those of 12 controls on a variety of psychometric measures as well as measures of body-size estimation, body satisfaction, and family interaction. No abnormalities in the parental attitudes toward weight control, body-size estimation, or body satisfaction were found, nor did the parents show any significant increase in psychopathology. On the family assessment measure, the anorectic families reported more difficulties on Task Accomplishment, Role Performance, Communication, and Affective Expression subscales than did the controls. Anorectics and their mothers scored lower on the Social Desirability scale. The investigators, however, were unable to determine if such disturbances were a part of the result or the cause of the illness. Three studies attempting to identify weight pathology in the parents of anorectics produced negative findings. Halmi, Struss, and Goldberg (1978) compared the weight of the parents of 30 anorectics with those of 30 normal controls and detected no difference between the two groups, although the investigators found higher educational level to be correlated with lower weight in the parents. Hall, Leibrich, Walkey, and Welch (1986), using a self-report questionnaire, found 58 mothers of anorectic patients to score the lowest on measures of weight pathology when compared to three control groups of mothers; they offer no explanation of this unexpected finding. Garfinkel, Garner, Rose, Darby, Brandes, O'Hanlon, and Walsh (1983) also found no difference in the parental weights of anorectics and controls when socioeconomic status was controlled.

The older literature generally described the mothers of anorectics as overprotective, intrusive, and dominating and the fathers as distant and passive (Kay & Leigh, 1954; King, 1963; Nemiah, 1950; Wall, 1959). Minuchin and his colleagues (Minuchin, Rosman, & Baker, 1978; Minuchin & Fishman, 1981), using a systems perspective, identified several characteristics of anorectic families: enmeshment, overprotectiveness, rigidity, conflict avoidance, and poor conflict resolution. More formal attempts to test these hypotheses have begun only recently. The issue is complicated by the fact that eating-disorder patients do not constitute a homogeneous group: The families of restrictive anorectics may interact very differently from those of bulimic anorectics or normal-weight bulimics. Using the Family Environment Scale (FES; Moos & Moos, 1980) Johnson and Flach (1985) studied 105 female normal-weight bulimics and 86 controls matched for various social and family variables. The bulimic patients perceived their families to be less cohesive; less open in expression of feelings; more conflictual; less encouraging of independence and assertiveness; less involved in intellectual, cultural, or recreational activities (although sharing high achievement expectations); and less concerned with moral and religious issues. Using the FES and the Family Adaptability and Cohesion Evaluation Scales (FACES; Olson, Bell, & Protner, 1978), Ordman and Kirschenbaum (1986) and Humphrey

(1986a) found similar results in normal-weight bulimics and bulimic anorectics. While the consistency of the findings is encouraging, the studies may be criticized for relying on the subjects' perception of their families. Using the Structural Analysis of Social Behavior (SASB; Benjamin, 1974), Humphrey (1987) directly studied the families (all intact) of 16 bulimic anorectics and 24 normal controls. The results indicated that the families of bulimic anorectics, when compared with their nondistressed counterparts, were more belittling, appeasing, ignoring, and walling-off as well as less helping, trusting, nurturing, and approaching. Again using the SASB, Humphrey (1986b) also studied the perceptions of four groups of subjects: normal-weight bulimics, bulimic anorectics, restrictive anorectics, and normal controls. The results indicated that bulimics, whether normal-weight or emaciated, reported not only greater family distress but also severe deficits in parental nurturance, understanding, and empathy. In contrast, the restrictive anorectics reported more family distress and hostility than controls but perceived their families as more affectionate than the bulimics. Humphrey concludes that the families of bulimics are more hostilely enmeshed and neglectful while those of restrictive anorectics are more "pseudo-mutual." Strober and colleagues (1982) found the families of bulimic anorectics to be more dissatisfied, conflictual, and negative, as well as less cohesive and organized, than those of restrictors. Furthermore, mothers of bulimic anorectics were more depressed and hostile and fathers of bulimics, more impulsive and irritable. Kog, Vandereycken, and Vertommen (1985), using a self-report questionnaire, found anorectic and bulimic families to have high enmeshment, but they were unable to clearly identify other characteristics, such as rigidity or conflict avoidance. In sum, disturbed family interaction is likely to be more common in eating-disorder families than normal families, and perhaps such disturbances are more overt in the families of bulimic patients than those of restrictive anorectics. Whether such patterns are pathognomonic of an eating disorder remains to be studied.

Many authors have suggested that the anorectic illness serves to stabilize the family environment. Different mechanisms have been proposed as to how this actually operates. The role of the family in the pathogenesis of the eating disorders will be discussed further in Chapter 4.

Finally, higher maternal age in anorexia nervosa patients has been reported by a number of investigators (Garfinkel & Garner, 1982; Hall, 1978; Halmi, Goldberg, Eckert, Casper, & Davis, 1977; Theander, 1970). However, Hare and Moran (1979) found older maternal and paternal age to be associated with *all* of the major psychiatric disorders, as compared to general population figures. It is therefore unlikely that older maternal age is specifically important for the pathogenesis of anorexia nervosa.

PHYSICAL SIGNS

Apart from the striking emaciation, positive signs are relatively uncommon in the restrictive anorectic. Some 50% of patients may have dry skin, sometimes with yellowish discoloration (possibly related to increased carotene deposition); lanugo over the trunk, face, and extremities; cold and cyanotic peripheries; dependent edema; bradycardia; and hypotension (Palla & Litt, 1988; Silverman, 1983). Osteopenia (bone loss) may occur resulting in pathological fractures (Rigotti, Nussbaum, Herzog, & Neer, 1984). Stunted growth may occur in patients with an early onset of anorexia nervosa, although with recovery, normal "catch-up" growth may occur (Pfeiffer, Lucas, & Ilstrup, 1986), presumably because the bone loss is reversible (Treasure, Russell, Fogelman, & Murby, 1987).

The bulimic patient may display swelling of the salivary (particularly the parotid) glands due to inflammation caused by the bingeing, vomiting, and perhaps excessive gum chewing; dental erosion; and callouses on the dorsum of the dominant hand caused by repeated abrasion of the skin by the incisors while inducing vomiting (Russell, 1979). If examined soon after a binge-and-vomit episode, the bulimic patient may appear flushed, and petechial hemorrhages may be seen on the cornea and the face. Chronic abuse of syrup of ipecac may cause generalized muscle pain and tenderness. Examination of the other systems is often negative unless the patient is in cardiac or renal failure. Anorexia nervosa has been reported to occur in subjects with Turner syndrome (Darby et al., 1981) or those with a hypothalamic tumor (Lewin, Mattingly, & Millis, 1972; Weller & Weller, 1982). A careful physical examination should always be made for an eating-disorder patient.

LABORATORY FINDINGS

Abnormal laboratory findings in the eating disorders occur as a result of (1) the starvation process, (2) the chaotic eating pattern, and (3) the use of substances to induce weight loss or decrease intake.

Starvation may lead to a normocytic normochromic anemia and leucopenia with relative lymphocytosis (Halmi, 1978). A low intake of foods containing iron folate may also contribute to anemia. A low erythrocyte sedimentation rate in anorexia nervosa distinguishes it from most of the other diseases that cause weight loss. Elevated blood levels of β-hydroxybutyric acid and free fatty acids occur as a result of the starvation, and these two findings are present in many apparently normal-weight bulimic patients (Pirke et al., 1985). Electrocardiographic changes, such as a low amplitude or sinus bradycardia, may occur, as well as impaired respiratory function (Keys et al., 1950). All these changes are readily reversible with nutritional replenishment.

Vomiting, laxative, and diuretic abuse cause hypokalemia, and sometimes hyponatremia as well if salt intake is low (patients sometimes avoid salt because they think it may lead to weight gain). Such electrolyte disturbances, as well as the loss of ventricular muscle, often lead to electrocardiographic changes. In a series of 65 preadolescent and adolescent anorectics and bulimics, gross electrocardiogram changes occurred in some 80% of the patients on admission (Palla & Litt, 1988). Proteinuria is common, but the cause is unclear. In some cases it may reflect excessive exercising. Chronic hypokalemia may cause renal damage and proteinuria. Inflammation of the salivary glands, due presumably to repeated vomiting, causes a rise in serum amylase (Mitchell, Pyle, Eckert, Hatsukami, & Lentz, 1983), sometimes mistaken for pancreatitis. Prolonged fasting may cause hypoglycemia. Patients sometimes ingest large quantities of carrots and green vegetables, which may lead to hypercarotenemia, while hypercholesterolemia may occur as a result of ingestion of high-cholesterol foods or perhaps the low calorie intake (Nestel, 1973). Ingestion of emetics, such as syrup of ipecac, causes myopathy, including cardiomyopathy. Iron deficiency anemia may occur if there is chronic laxative abuse that leads to rectal bleeding.

Electroencephalographic changes occur in some 40% to 50% of patients (Crisp, Fenton, & Scotton, 1968; Neil et al., 1980), more frequently in bulimics than restrictors. The significance of the 14- and 6-per-second positive spiking in bulimia (Rau & Green, 1984) is unclear, but it is apparently unrelated to response to anticonvulsants (Kaplan, 1987b). There has been speculation that the EEG changes are related to the fluid and electrolyte disturbances that occur in anorexia nervosa and bulimia nervosa (Crisp, 1980). Epileptic seizures may occur. The sleep EEGs of anorectics are characteristic of those with a chronic physical illness (Neil et al., 1980). Katz and colleagues (Katz et al., 1984) found the sleep EEGs of anorectics to resemble those of major depressives, particularly with respect to shortened REM (rapid-eye-movement sleep) latency, which is considered to be a biological marker for major depression (Gillin, Duncan, Pettigrew, Frankel, & Snyder, 1979; Kupfer, Foster, Reich, Thompson, & Weiss, 1976). However, at least four other groups of investigators have been unable to replicate these findings (Hudson, Pope, Jonas, Lipinski, & Kupfer, 1987; Levy, Dixon, & Schmidt, 1987; Neil et al., 1980; Walsh, Goetz, Roose, Fingeroth, & Glassman, 1985). The sleep EEGs of normal-weight bulimics are essentially normal and do not resemble those of major depression (Hudson, Pope, Jonas, Yurgelun-Todd, & Frankenburg, 1987; Levy et al., 1987; Walsh et al., 1985). Cerebral atrophy is found on computerized tomography scans but is apparently reversible with weight gain (Krieg, Pirke, Laver, & Backmund, 1988; Nussbaum, Shenker, Marc, & Klein, 1980). The many medical complications of the two disorders are summarized in Tables 2.2 and 2.3. In summary, clinicians taking care of anorectic and bulimic patients should be well aware of the potentially serious physical complications that may occur in these patients.

ENDOCRINE DISTURBANCES IN ANOREXIA NERVOSA

The endocrine disturbances that occur in anorexia nervosa have most often been compared to those that occur in nonanorectic starvation states and in major depression. The endocrine changes in anorexia nervosa are largely, although not entirely, a product of starvation, and the hope of finding an endocrinological cause for the illness or linking the illness to the affective disorders has so far not materialized. The following account is a simplified summary of the current findngs. Interested readers should refer to the major recent reviews (Fava,

TABLE 2.2. Medical Complications in Restrictive Anorexia Nervosa

Findings	Possible mechanisms	Clinical significance
Endocrine		
Amenorrhea, polycystic ovaries	Probably related to self-imposed starvation, exact mechanisms unclear	Usually reversible with weight gain and normalization of eating habits and mood
Blunted LH response to LHRH		
Low T3 and T4		
Growth hormone, prolactin, somatomedin and somatostatin, norepinephrine, cortisol, arginine vasopressin, and other disturbances		
Metabolic		
Electrolytes usually normal but may show low potassium, low sodium, low chloride, high or low bicarbonate	Starvation	May lead to cardiac arrest, chronic changes may lead to and are signs of renal failure; specific treatment needed
Osteoporosis and retarded bone growth	Malnutrition	Short stature; pathological fractures
Low cholesterol	Malnutrition	Unclear
High cholesterol	Unclear, maybe related to dietary imbalance	Unclear
Hypercarotenemia	Unclear	Unclear
Abnormal glucose tolerance	? starvation	Unclear
Abnormal temperature regulation	? starvation	Unclear
High β-hydroxybutyric acid	Starvation	Improves with recovery
High free fatty acids		

(continued)

TABLE 2.2. *(continued)*

Findings	Possible mechanisms	Clinical significance
Cardiovascular		
Bradycardia	Starvation	Improves with recovery
Hypotension	Starvation	Improves with recovery
Heart failure	Starvation and electrolyte imbalance	May lead to death; specific treatment needed
EKG changes	Starvation and electrolyte imbalance	May be indications of heart failure or electrolyte imbalance
Peripheral edema	Starvation, electrolyte imbalance, possible rapid refeeding	Monitor renal and cardiac function; may need specific treatment
Pulmonary		
Changes in pulmonary function	Starvation	Unclear
Gastrointestinal		
Constipation	Starvation	Improves with recovery
Decreased gastric emptying	? starvation	Improves with recovery, causes subjective distress
Acute gastric dilatation	? rapid feeding	May lead to death; specific treatment needed
Increased hepatic enzymes	? starvation	Improves with recovery

Renal		
Low blood urea nitrogen	Starvation	Improves with recovery
Increased blood urea nitrogen	Renal function impairment unusual unless purging	A sign of renal failure; may need specific treatment
Decreased glomerular filtration rate (e.g., low creatinine)	Renal function impairment unusual unless purging	A sign of renal failure; may need specific treatment
See also metabolic changes		
Neurological		
Epileptic seizures	? starvation and electrolyte imbalance	May need specific treatment
CT scan changes	Starvation	Improves with recovery
EEG and sleep EEG changes (conflicting)	Possibly related to starvation	Unclear
Hematologic		
Anemia	Starvation	Improves with recovery
Pancytopenia		
Bone marrow hypocellularity		
Thrombcytopenia		
Musculocutaneous		
Muscle weakening	Electrolyte imbalance	Improves with correction of electrolyte imbalance and malnutrition
Lanugo hair	Starvation	Improves with recovery
Cold extremities	Starvation	Improves with recovery

45

TABLE 2.3. Medical Complications in Bulimia Nervosa

Findings	Possible mechanisms	Clinical significance
Endocrine		
Menstrual irregularity	Probably malnutrition	Unusually reversible with recovery
Other endocrine disturbances similar to anorexia nervosa may be present		
Metabolic		
Low potassium	Vomiting, laxative and/or diuretic abuse	May lead to cardiac arrest and renal failure; may be a sign of renal failure; specific treatment needed.
Low sodium		
Low chloride		
High or low bicarbonate		
Other metabolic disturbances similar to anorexia nervosa may be present		
Cardiovascular		
Cardiomyopathy	Ipecac abuse	May lead to death
Heart failure	Electrolyte disturbance, ipecac abuse	May lead to death; specific treatment needed
EKG changes	Electrolyte disturbance, cardiomyopathy, heart failure	May be indication of heart failure or cardiomyopathy
Peripheral edema	Usually from rebound fluid retention after purging	Monitor cardiac and renal function
Pulmonary		
Aspiration pneumonia	Aspiration of vomitus	May need specific treatment

Gastrointestinal		
Gastric and duodenal ulcer	Binge-eating and vomiting	May need specific treatment
Decreased gastric emptying	? starvation	Improves with recovery
Acute gastric dilatation, parotid swelling	Binge-eating	May lead to death; specific treatment needed
Increased amylase	? parotid inflammation from vomiting	Improves with recovery
Renal		
Low blood urea nitrogen	Starvation	Improves with recovery
High blood urea nitrogen	Renal function impairment, usually result of chronic purging	Sign of renal failure
Decreased glomerular filtration	Renal function impairment, usually result of purging	Sign of renal failure
Neurological		
Epileptic seizures	? malnutrition and electrolyte imbalance	May need specific treatment
EEG & sleep EEG changes (conflicting)	Unclear	Unclear
Hematologic		
Anemia	Dietary deficiency	May need supplements
Musculocutaneous		
Muscle weakening	Electrolyte imbalance, ipecac abuse	Correction of underlying problems
Callouses on dorsum of dominant hand	Repeated abrasion	None

Copeland, Schweiger, & Herzog, 1989; Isaacs, 1979; Wakeling, 1985; Walsh, 1982; Weiner, 1983).

Hypothalamic–Pituitary–Ovarian (HPO) Axis

Normally the hypothalamus produces luteinizing hormone–releasing hormone (LHRH), which stimulates the pituitary to secrete luteinizing hormone (LH) and follicle-stimulating hormone (FSH). These hormones then stimulate the ovaries to produce estrogen and progesterone; estrogen in turn exerts both positive and negative feedback effects on both the pituitary and hypothalamus to regulate the ovulatory and menstrual functions in a normal female.

In anorexia nervosa there is a deficiency in the secretion of LHRH, leading to low levels of both the pituitary gonadotropins and ovarian hormones. Thus the amenorrhea in anorexia nervosa is due to a hypogonadotropic hypogonadism; that is, a decrease in the functioning of the entire hypothalamic–pituitary–ovarian axis. It is unclear what causes the deficient hypothalamic secretion of LHRH, although low body weight is a major factor. It is possible that psychological factors, such as weight phobia and depression, may also play a part.

In anorexia nervosa the pituitary gland has a low reserve of the gonadotropins LH and FSH, but this is reversible with weight gain. This low reserve may occur for two reasons: the already mentioned deficient LHRH secretion by the hypothalamus or an increased sensitivity to negative feedback of estrogens at low body weight. The positive feedback response of the pituitary to estrogens usually occurs with the restoration of normal weight; but it may take time, and such delayed recovery is probably the main reason for the persistent amenorrhea in some normal-weight patients. Theoretically it is possible to bypass the hypothalamus and the inhibitory feedback of estrogens by prolonged parenteral administration of synthetic LHRH, and the pituitary, even at low body weight, can then be stimulated to synthesize and secrete LH and FSH. In fact, several low-weight anorectics have actually been treated with prolonged LHRH infusion, and one patient became pregnant even though her body weight was very low (Nillius & Wide, 1977). The value of such treatments is obviously very questionable.

In the normal adult female, LH and FSH are secreted in a pulsatile fashion throughout the 24 hours. In children, basal LH and

FSH levels are very low and the fluctuations in the levels are very minor. In puberty, such pulsatile secretions are augmented during sleep, and the daytime levels of LH and FSH gradually increase until the adult pattern is established. In low-weight anorectics, the gonadotropin secretory pattern is either prepubertal or occurs early in puberty, and the pattern matures with weight gain. The LH response to stimulation by a bolus intravenous injection of synthetic LHRH is largely dependent on body weight. At low weight the response is minimal, but it increases with weight gain. However, FSH response may initially be exaggerated. Some studies have found a threshold weight of about 46 kilograms at which the LH and FSH responses are both exaggerated (Beumont, Abraham, & Turtle, 1980; Warren, 1977). As already mentioned, if LHRH is given repeatedly in a pulsatile manner instead of a single bolus injection, the pituitary even at low body weight will eventually produce a normal circadian LH pattern.

Stimulation of the pituitary can also be evoked by administration of clomiphene, a synthetic estrogen, which occupies the estrogen receptor sites at the hypothalamus and thus blocks the inhibitory feedback effect of estrogen on the hypothalamus. In anorectics clomiphene usually induces an increase in LH levels only when the patients are above 80% of average weight.

Anorectic patients metabolize estradiol, the main ovarian estrogen, differently from normal women. Instead of producing estriol, they produce more 2-OH estrone, which is much less active biologically. This 2-OH estrone essentially acts as an antiestrogen by occupying the estrogen receptors and perhaps also by inhibiting the secretion of LHRH. Again, weight gain normalizes this metabolic aberration. In summary, the dysfunction of the HPO axis in anorexia nervosa is mainly due to weight loss and malnutrition and is usually reversible with weight gain. To the best of my knowledge, the HPO axis function has not been studied in major depression.

Hypothalamic–Pituitary–Adrenal (HPA) Axis

In contrast to the diminished activity of the HPO axis, the activity of the hypothalamic–pituitary–adrenal axis is elevated in anorexia nervosa. Plasma cortisol levels are increased, and the normal diurnal variation in cortisol level is lost. In addition there is dexamethasone nonsuppression and decreased cortisol response to insulin hypoglycemia. These changes are in part due to an increased half-life of cortisol, which also occurs in starvation from other causes, and in part to a greater adrenal production of cortisol relative to the patient's body size. This greater cortisol production is probably due to an increase in the pituitary secretion of adrenal corticotropin (ACTH), which in turn is due to an increased hypothalamic secretion of corticotropin-releasing factor (CRF). The decreased metabolism of cortisol can be corrected by weight gain or the administration of triiodothyronine (T-3), which is low in both anorexia nervosa and starvation from other causes. The increased activation of the HPA axis resembles that in major depression but is opposite to what apparently occurs in malnutrition from other causes. However, it is readily reversible with even a small amount of weight gain.

In summary, the disturbances in the HPA axis in anorexia nervosa in part resemble those that occur in malnutrition from other causes and those that are found in major depression. The exact mechanisms of the disturbances are unclear.

Hypothalamic–Pituitary–Thyroid (HPT) Axis

In normal subjects the pituitary releases thyroid-stimulating hormone (TSH) in response to the thyrotropin-releasing hormone (TRH) secreted by the hypothalamus. The TSH stimulates the thyroid to produce thyroxine (T-4) and triiodothyronine (T-3), which then exert negative feedback effects on the pituitary. Patients with anorexia nervosa have a below-normal plasma level of T-4 and a markedly decreased plasma level of T-3. In addition, they exhibit several features characteristic of hypothyroidism, including cold intolerance, bradycardia, constipation, dry skin and hair, slow-relaxing reflexes, and low basal metabolic rate. However, the TSH level in anorectics is normal, and its response to an infusion of TRH is also normal, although the peak response may be significantly delayed. Such findings suggest that the anorectic patient is not truly suffering from hypothyroidism. The low T-3 probably results from a reduction in its peripheral conversion from T-4, a process that also occurs in starvation from other causes and is associated with an increased conversion of T-4 to inactive reverse T-3. These findings are different from those seen in patients with major depression and represent an adaptive response to starvation by reducing catabolism to conserve energy.

Growth Hormone and Prolactin

Growth hormone (GH) levels are often elevated in anorexia nervosa, secondary to reduced levels of somatomedin C. This seems to be secondary to the starvation state, and, even before any substantial weight gain occurs, normal levels appear with increased caloric intake. GH responses to provocative tests—such as the use of glucose loading, bromocriptine mesylate, and TRH—have been reported as impaired. This suggests a disturbance in the central mechanisms controlling GH release, but such disturbances are usually reversible with weight gain. The normal rise in GH during sleep is apparently retained in anorexia nervosa.

Hyperprolactinemia is associated with amenorrhea. In anorexia nervosa, however, prolactin levels are usually normal. Nocturnal prolactin levels are low and prolactin response to TRH is impaired in anorexia nervosa, but again these changes are usually reversible with weight gain.

Arginine Vasopressin

Defects in urinary concentration or dilution suggestive of abnormal secretion of the antidiuretic hormone, arginine vasopressin, have repeatedly been demonstrated in anorexia nervosa. Such defects are related either to a simple deficiency of vasopressin secretion or, more commonly, to erratic fluctuations in plasma levels of the hormone that bear no apparent relation to changes in plasma levels of sodium. Furthermore, the average concentration of arginine vasopressin in the cerebrospinal fluid (CSF) of anorectic patients varies much more from the mean than it does in normal subjects; indeed, the normal CSF/plasma ratio of arginine vasopressin is reversed. This abnormal osmoregulation of arginine vasopressin is not immediately corrected by improvement of weight and nutritional status, but, after a few months of normal-weight maintenance, it does revert to normal. The significance of these changes is unclear. They may reflect primary alterations in catecholamine metabolism, or they may be secondary to the patients' self-induced vomiting.

Gastrointestinal Hormones

There has been some renewed interest recently in the changes in the gastrointestinal functioning in eating disorders (Craigen, Kennedy, Garfinkel, & Jeejeebhoy, 1987; for normal physiology, see Guyton, 1986). Briefly, normal gastric emptying is regulated by a complex interplay of a host of factors that operate through two basic mechanisms: the nervous system (primarily the vagus nerve) and the gastrointestinal hormonal system. For instance, the vagus nerve stimulates the release of the hormone gastrin, which increases gastric emptying; the gastric contents that are emptied in turn stimulate, via chemoreceptors in the duodenal wall, the release of hormones such as secretin, gastric inhibitory peptide, and cholecystokinin, which then inhibit gastric emptying. The content and acidity of the chyme also regulate the rate of gastric emptying; for instance, high-fat and high-protein foods as well as high-acidity chyme slow gastric emptying. Finally, certain hormones that are secreted by the brain, such as TRH and ACTH, are also secreted by the gut. The role of such gut hormones is, however, unclear.

In anorexia nervosa and bulimia nervosa there is delayed gastric emptying of solid foods and perhaps also of liquids. The reason for this delay is unclear, but it may be linked to a disturbance in neurohormonal controls. Clinical experience suggests that this disturbance, commonly reported as abdominal fullness and distension even after a small meal, improves with weight gain.

Central Nervous System Neurotransmitters

Recent studies indicate that hypothalamic neurotransmitter systems may be involved in the control of eating behavior in animals and humans (Fava et al., 1989; Leibowitz & Shor-Posner, 1986). In addition, central nervous system neurotransmitters may play a role in the pathogenesis of psychiatric disorders such as depression, anxiety, schizophrenia, and obsessive–compulsive disorder. For the eating disorders, at least three neurotransmitters have been implicated: serotonin (5-HT), norepinephrine (NE), and dopamine (DA). The classical notion that the medial hypothalamus functions as the satiety center while the lateral hypothalamus acts as the feeding center no longer stands, although with their abundant innervation with serotonergic, adrenergic, noradrenergic, and dopaminergic neurons and receptors, the hypothalamus most probably functions as an integrating center for various inputs of feeding and satiety.

The first indication that 5-HT was involved in the control of feeding was probably the finding that serotonergic agonists caused a reduction in food intake in animals and humans. These 5-HT agonists include 5-HT uptake blockers (such as fluoxetine and chlorimipramine) and agents (such as fenfluramine), which enhance the presynaptic release of 5-HT. Further studies in animals involved the injection of serotonergic agents directly into the brain, particularly into the hypothalamus. Infusion of serotonergic agents to the medial hypothalamus is followed by suppression of eating in the animal, in particular a decrease in the duration and size of the meal; that is, a satiety effect. Furthermore, it seems that the animal rather specifically decreases the proportion of carbohydrates in the meal.

In contrast, infusion of NE into the medial hypothalamus causes an increase in meal size and duration as well as a specific preference for carbohydrates. This NE-stimulated eating is inhibited by 5-HT and other serotonergic agents. Dopamine seems to act via the lateral hypothalamus to produce a decrease in feeding by delaying meal onset, in contrast to the satiety effect of 5-HT. DA blockers, such as chlorpromazine and haloperidol, have the opposite effect, while amphetamine is believed to exert its nonspecific anorectic effect through the activation of the lateral hypothalamic dopaminergic neurons.

The central nervous system synthesis of these neurotransmitters is in turn influenced by the dietary composition and the animal's temporal feeding pattern. A high-carbohydrate meal causes an increase in plasma tryptophan and subsequently brain tryptophan, which, being a precursor of 5-HT, eventually produces an increase in the brain 5-HT as well. A high-protein diet, however, decreases the entry of tryptophan to the brain (through the increased synthesis of other amino acids that compete with tryptophan for entry into the brain) and thus eventually causes a decrease in brain 5-HT. Thus neurotransmitters in the brain may determine food choices, which in turn determine the brain levels of neurotransmitters.

However, it must be stated that the findings reviewed above are very preliminary. The control of eating behavior in humans is obviously complex, involving a variety of psychosocial as well as biological events. Indirect methods of measuring central nervous system neurotransmitters in humans are fraught with problems since their levels are influenced by many factors, some of which are difficult to control at this stage of our knowledge. The following account is a brief summary of recent findings: In anorexia nervosa, the plasma tryptophan level and its ratio to the other large neutral amino acids that compete with it for entrance to the brain are both low. The 5-hydroxyindoleacetic acid (5-HIAA), a metabolite of 5-HT, is also low in the CSF of underweight anorectics, particularly bulimic anorectics. The CSF 5-HIAA levels seem to increase with partial weight restoration (Kaye, Gwirstman, George, Jimerson, & Ebert, 1988). If confirmed, these findings may indicate a deficit of 5-HT functioning in the brain in some anorectics, or perhaps simply a decrease in carbohydrate intake.

As already mentioned, dopamine injection to the lateral hypothalamus decreases eating, and Barry and Klawans (1976) have speculated that increased cerebral dopaminergic activity might account for the symptoms of anorexia nervosa. However, CSF levels of the dopamine metabolite, homovanillic acid, in underweight anorectics have been found to be either low or not different from normals (for a review, see Fava et al., 1989). The use of dopamine blocking agents, such as pimozide, in anorexia nervosa is not effective (Vandereycken, 1987).

Low CSF and peripheral (plasma or urinary) concentrations of 3-methoxy-4-hydroxy phenylglycol (MHPG), a metabolite of norepinephrine, occurs in anorexia nervosa (Biederman et al., 1984; Halmi, Dekirmenjian, Davis, Casper, & Goldberg, 1978). Low MHPG excretion has also been reported in some depressives. CSF norepinephrine levels have been found to be low in underweight anorectics, although they normalize after nutritional rehabilitation (Gerner et al., 1984; Kaye, Ebert, Raleigh, & Lake, 1984). However, lower CSF norepinephrine levels may persist in some apparently weight-recovered anorectics. If confirmed, this finding may indicate impaired NE metabolism in anorexia nervosa.

Finally, opioid peptide may be involved in the control of eating behavior (Morley & Levine, 1980; Sanger, 1981). However, there are numerous opioid peptides (Bloom, 1983), and the role of each in the control of eating behavior may be quite distinct. Thus, perhaps not surprisingly, attempts to measure opioid activity in anorexia nervosa have produced conflicting results (Kaye, 1987).

ENDOCRINE DISTURBANCES IN BULIMIA NERVOSA

The endocrine disturbances in bulimia nervosa have not been studied extensively. Current findings may be summarized as follows.

Hypothalamic–Pituitary–Adrenal Axis

Cortisol levels and 24-hour cortisol secretion patterns are normal in bulimia nervosa. Dexamethasone suppression test in bulimia is often abnormal, but the significance of this finding is unclear, since it is not related to duration or severity of illness or to presence or absence of concurrent depression (for a review, see Walsh, Roose, Lindy, Gladis, & Glassman, 1987).

Hypothalamic–Pituitary–Ovarian Axis

As already mentioned, menstrual irregularity and amenorrhea are common in apparently normal-weight bulimic women. Cystic ovarian changes that occur in anorexia nervosa also occur in some bulimic patients (Treasure, 1988). Estradiol levels, which normally parallel the development of the follicle in the ovary, and progesterone levels, which parallel development of the corpus luteum, are low in many bulimics. The 24-hour LH and FSH levels are also low in many bulimics, particularly those of FSH. Despite the fact that patients who demonstrate these abnormalities are within normal weight range, their body weight as a group is significantly lower than those whose hormonal levels are normal. Thus strict dieting and a state of semi-starvation may be responsible for such hormonal changes (Pirke et al., 1987).

Hypothalamic–Pituitary–Thyroid Axis

Overall, recent research has found that bulimic patients in general have normal thyroxine (T-4) and triiodothyronine (T-3) levels. However, T-3 levels may sometimes be significantly lower than normal among bulimics who are at a low average weight (Pirke et al., 1987). This finding is generally interpreted to mean that the patients may be biologically starved even though they are at a relatively normal weight. Recently, studies in depression of TSH response to TRH have stimulated similar studies in bulimia nervosa. A blunted TSH response to TRH, considered to be a characteristic of major depression, is found also in some normal-weight bulimic patients, but apparently not more commonly than in normal controls (Kaplan, 1987a; Levy, Dixon, & Malarkey, 1988). However, Levy and colleagues (1988) found

TRH to produce abnormally high prolactin and growth hormone responses. These investigators suggest that such abnormal responses to TRH may indicate a neuroendocrine abnormality in this disorder.

Central Nervous System Opioids, Catecholamines, and Serotonin

The data here are conflicting. No definite abnormality in any of these neurotransmitters has been found, except perhaps for a low norepinephrine level. Opiate antagonists (such as naloxone) and serotonin agonists (such as fluoxetine) appear to be useful for decreasing bulimic episodes in bulimia nervosa (for reviews, see Jimerson, George, Kaye, Brewerton, & Goldstein, 1987; Mitchell, Morley, Levine, & Hatsukami, 1987).

Cholecystokinin

Cholecystokinin is an intestinal hormone released after eating that normally promotes satiety. In a pilot study of 14 bulimics, Geracioti and Liddle (1988) found an impaired cholecystokinin response to eating. After an open trial of antidepressants in a subgroup of five patients, the postprandial cholecystokinin response normalized, accompanied by increased subjective satiety. The findings are intriguing and obviously need further study, possibly with, for instance, the rate of gastric emptying (which affects cholecystokinin secretion) properly controlled for (Herzog & Copeland, 1988).

EATING DISORDERS IN THE MALE

The occurrence of anorexia nervosa in the male was recognized by both Morton (1694) and Gull (1874). Recently several studies on relatively large numbers of male anorectics have been reported (Andersen, 1985; Burns & Crisp, 1984; Crisp & Toms, 1972; Hasan & Tibbetts, 1977). From the case material presented, it would appear that the clinical features and outcome of anorexia nervosa in the male are essentially similar to those in the female (Crisp, Burns, & Bhat,

1986). Of course, amenorrhea does not occur in the male, but male anorectics frequently have low or absent sexual interest or drive. Andersen (1985) holds the view that the clinical picture for the male is different from that for the female, but he does not elaborate. He suggests that male anorectics be divided into three groups according to age of onset: prepubertal, adolescent, and adult. However, the same classification can apply to female patients, and it cannot therefore be held to indicate a difference between male and female patients. Needless to say, the precipitating factors are likely to be different for males, but, then, even for females there are no illness-specific precipitating factors other than the dieting behavior. Andersen's view that adolescent-onset male anorectics are more often obese and have greater sexual identity conflicts is intriguing but needs to be substantiated. In terms of endocrine findings, the few endocrine studies that have been published found that levels of LH, FSH, and testosterone are low during the low-weight phase of the illness but that these levels increase with weight gain (Crisp, Hsu, Chen, & Wheeler, 1982). Again, there seems to be a threshold weight at which paradoxical LH and FSH responses to LHRH occur.

Two studies on relatively large numbers of male bulimics have recently been published (Mitchell & Goff, 1984; Schneider & Agras, 1987). Again, the clinical features in males and females appear to be very similar. Schneider and Agras (1987) found a higher prevalence of homosexual or bisexual preference and more problems with drugs and alcohol among the males than the females.

Various authors have speculated on why the eating disorders are relatively rare among the males (Andersen, 1985; Crisp & Toms, 1972; Scott, 1987). My hypothesis is that it is directly related to the fact that fewer males than females diet to control or lose weight (see Chapter 4). Furthermore, perhaps males are less bothered by fatness, since they increase in muscularity rather than fat during puberty and, in contrast to adolescent females, adolescent males often want to be bigger and taller. The factors that intensify dieting in the adolescent female, such as poor body concept, self-esteem, and identity confusion, do not seem to affect the adolescent male as much, or at least they do not usually drive him to go on a diet. Finally, eating disorders in the male are perhaps underdiagnosed and underreported, since they are commonly assumed to be female disorders; they are also easier to disguise because of the way men dress.

CONCLUSION

In this chapter we have reviewed the clinical features of anorexia nervosa and bulimia nervosa. The illnesses commonly begin in adolescence and affect females much more than males. However, the clinical features are not remarkably different when the illnesses occur in older females or in males. Many of the patients' symptoms and behaviors occur directly as a result of starvation. Family studies have found a preponderance of major affective illnesses and eating disorders in first- and second-degree relatives. Biological studies have found, in general, that the identified neuroendocrine and metabolic disturbances are secondary to the starvation.

Many popular clinical impressions, such as those regarding personality characteristics or family interactions, have not been subjected to critical study, and the studies that have been done often result in conflicting findings. Clearly, better research strategies are needed to study the psychosocial aspects of the disorders. No doubt more intensive biological research will continue, and one hopes that, with improved basic techniques, the biological disturbances in the disorders will be clarified.

3

Epidemiology

Epidemiological studies have confirmed the clinical impression that the eating disorders are more prevalent among young Caucasian females from the middle to upper social classes in Western cultures. They have also suggested that the incidence of anorexia nervosa may be increasing in the developed countries and that immigrants from other cultures tend to develop abnormal eating attitudes and behavior as they become acculturated. Furthermore, while hard data are lacking, there is a strong impression that the eating disorders are rare in developing countries, but become more common as a country develops economically. Finally, the same factors that characterize eating-disorder patients also characterize the population that is most concerned about dieting, weight, and shape.

The purpose of epidemiological studies is, narrowly speaking, to provide statistics concerning the extent (i.e., distribution, incidence, prevalence, and duration) of morbidity in a population, to relate it to the environment of the population, to detect its association with possible causative factors, and to determine the resources required to deal with such morbidity. Epidemiological figures are most often expressed in incidence and prevalence rates. The term *incidence* refers to the number of new cases that appear in a defined community within a specified time period (usually 1 year), most commonly expressed as the rate per 100,000 of the population. *Prevalence* refers to the actual number of cases in a defined community at a point in time. Rates are "crude" if the figures have not been adjusted for other variables, such as age or sex. In the case of the epidemiology of eating disorders, we are primarily at the stage of determining the incidence and prevalence rates of the disorders within populations and comparing the rates among different population groups. As such, we grapple mainly with two methodological issues: The definition of a case of eating disorder and the detection of the number of cases within a specified population. However, a few studies are beginning to explore possible causative factors associated with the development of the eating disorders. This chapter reviews the case record and questionnaire studies, the two-stage studies, and the recent high-risk studies as well as epidemiological studies of dieting behavior. I then state my hypothesis that abnormal eating behaviors occur on a continuum occupied on the one end by simple dieting and on the other by diagnosable eating disorders.

DEFINITION OF A CASE

At first sight the definitions of anorexia nervosa and bulimia nervosa appear straightforward. However, if we use a clinically useful definition (such as the *DSM-III-R* criteria) to identify a case, we may exclude the "subclinical" cases that show only a "partial syndrome" and thus obtain an incomplete picture of the extent of morbidity in the community. The amount of weight loss, duration of amenorrhea, and frequency of bingeing and purging are quantitative phenomena, and the choice of a cutoff between a "case" and a "noncase" is therefore arbitrary and related largely to the purpose of the study (Copeland, 1981). For instance, it may be appropriate to use strict criteria for a study designed to determine the number of hospital beds required for the treatment of the eating disorders, while a broader definition may be more appropriate for a study designed to determine the relation of the illness to sociocultural variables (Szmukler, 1985). In my view, it is important that both the diagnosable and subclinical cases be reported in studies designed to elucidate causative factors, so that we can understand what factors determine the expression of symptoms and how the severity of symptoms may change over time.

Because the eating disorders are comparatively rare, large populations must be studied to gain an accurate figure for the incidence of the disorders. This poses tremendous difficulties for case detection, since direct interviews by trained researchers are not feasible. Thus far investigators have used two approaches to circumvent this difficulty. The first is to rely on hospital records and case registers, and the second is to use a two-stage process of case identification.

CASE REGISTER AND
HOSPITAL RECORD STUDIES

Epidemiological studies using hospital records or case registers base their definition of a case on the clinician's diagnosis. However, clinicians do not always use well-defined diagnostic criteria, and in the seven studies listed in Table 3.1 only Lucas, Beard, O'Fallon, and Kurland (1988), Theander (1970), and Willi and Grossman (1983) used explicitly stated criteria that included weight loss, food refusal, and amenorrhea. Szmukler and colleagues (1985), in applying Russell's (1970) criteria to a sample of patients listed on the Aberdeen (Scotland) Case Register, found that only 23% of the case notes examined had recorded all of Russell's three criteria: 57% had recorded two; 15%, one; and 5%, none. Thus diagnostic differences among studies must have accounted for at least some of the discrepancies in the findings. Furthermore, since some studies used hospital records that included only inpatients, while others used case registers that included all new contacts with psychiatric treatment agencies, this difference in patient selection also undoubtedly contributed to the variation in the findings among studies.

The limitations of case register studies are considerable. By including only patients who enter the psychiatric health care system, they fail to detect those who are under the care of nonpsychiatric systems. Jones, Fox, Babigan, and Hutton (1980) and Szmukler, McCance, McCrone, and Hunter (1986) found that the case registers of Monroe County, New York and northeast Scotland failed to record about 13% of all the cases in either area. Combining case registers with hospital records may help overcome a part of this difficulty but will still leave out those who have never entered a health care system. Given the secretive nature of the eating disorders, the number of "cases" who have never sought medical consultation for their eating

TABLE 3.1. Incidence of Anorexia Nervosa by Case Registers and Hospital Records

Study	Source	Diagnostic criteria	Region	Period	Incidence per 100,000 per year[b]
Hoek & Brook (1985)	Case register	—	Groningen	1974–1982	5.0
Jones et al. (1980)	Both	Weight loss and anorexia for hospital cases	Monroe County	1970–1976	0.64 (Caucasians only)
Kendell et al. (1973)	Case register	—	Camberwell, Monroe County, NE Scotland	1965–1960 1960–1969 1966–1969	0.66 0.37 1.60
Lucas et al. (1988)	Both	Russell's criteria primarily (see text)	Rochester, Minnesota	1935–1979	7.3 overall 56.7 for females (age 15–19)
Szmukler et al. (1986)	Case register	See text	NE Scotland	1978–1982	4.06 4.68[a] 30 (age 16–25) 50 (age 18)
Theander (1970)	Hospital record	Pursuit of thinness, amenorrhea, weight loss	Southern Sweden	1933–1960 1951–1960	0.24 0.45
Willi & Grossman (1983)	Hospital record	Weight loss, amenorrhea, food refusal (ages 12–25)	Zurich	1956–1958 1963–1965 1973–1975	0.38 0.55 1.12

[a]If both case register and hospital records are used.
[b]Females only.

62

disorder may be considerable. Finally, all the studies focused only on anorexia nervosa, probably because bulimia nervosa was considered a variant of anorexia nervosa until the late 1970s. The Mayo Clinic study (Lucas et al., 1988) has overcome several of these difficulties. The period of study (1935–1979) was lengthy. The geographical area was well-defined, and the Mayo Clinic records contained practically all medical contacts for individuals living in Rochester, Minnesota. The diagnostic criteria used were basically equivalent to the *DSM-III-R* criteria for anorexia nervosa. All records of patients with a clinical diagnosis of anorexia nervosa and those with amenorrhea were screened, as well as a representative proportion of all records showing weight loss, endocrine dysfunction, or abnormal eating behaviors and attitudes. The findings of this study are therefore particularly significant, although some of its conclusions are open to dispute, which we will discuss later.

All the studies showed that anorexia nervosa primarily affects young women, with a peak incidence around the age of 18. All except the Mayo Clinic study found that the incidence of the disorder has been increasing in recent years. However, the increase in incidence of the disorder has occurred primarily among women between the ages of 15 and 24; there has been little or no increase for women in other age categories or for men. In the two areas where mixed ethnic groups were studied (Monroe County, New York and Camberwell, London), non-Caucasian patients were rare. A preponderance of patients from the higher social classes was found in all areas except for northeast Scotland and Monroe County in the study by Kendell, Hall, Hailey, and Babigian (1973). However, the influence of social class on the incidence of the illness may not be straightforward. While there appeared to be no correlation between incidence and social class in northeast Scotland and Monroe County in the 1960s, such an association was established in both areas by the two later studies of Jones and colleagues (1980) and Szmukler and colleagues (1985). Furthermore, this correlation between social class and incidence of illness did not apply to the younger patients in Monroe County (Jones et al., 1980), and Szmukler and colleagues (1986) found an underrepresentation of Social Class III (i.e., middle class) among patients in northeast Scotland. Thus socioeconomic factors appear to operate through other intervening variables. As already mentioned, the Mayo Clinic study (Lucas et al., 1988) has distinct advantages over the other studies.

Because of the careful screening and the availability of more complete and consistent medical records, it is not surprising that the incidence rates in the Mayo Clinic study were much higher than those in other studies. The overall annual incidence rate in this study was 8.2 per 100,000, 13.5 for females, and 1.6 for males. The highest age-specific incidence rate, 56.7 per 100,000, occurred in females 15- to 19-years-old. The prevalence rate on January 1, 1980, for this age group was 1 in 332 (about 0.3%). In contrast to the other studies, the Mayo Clinic study found no consistent increase in incidence among females in recent years (incidences in males were too low in all the studies to allow for any meaningful interpretation). Instead, it found low incidence rates for 1950–1964 and higher rates for 1935–1949 and 1965–1979. The authors suggest that perhaps different sociocultural inferences had caused the variation in the incidence rates. If so, it may be that only young women are susceptible to such influences, since this change in incidence rates occurred primarily in women who were 10- to 19-years-old, while the rate for women who were 20- to 59-years-old remained remarkably similar during the 45 years of the study.

However, these conclusions may be open to dispute. Andersen (1988) has pointed out that if the probable and possible cases are excluded, the data might have shown an increase in the definite cases. Lucas (personal communication, November 1989) has recently extended the Mayo Clinic study to include data up to 1984 and found, as in the other studies, a definite increase in incidence of the disorder in women aged 15 to 24 over the 50-year period of the study (1935–1984). The evidence from the case record studies indicates that the incidence of anorexia nervosa seems to be increasing in Western countries.

QUESTIONNAIRE AND INTERVIEW STUDIES

To overcome the limitations of case register and hospital record studies, researchers have adopted other approaches to survey the population for the incidence of eating disorders. Crisp, Palmer, and Kalucy (1976) surveyed nine schools, seven private and two state-run, by interviewing the teachers and, in an unspecified proportion of cases, also the students. They found an incidence of 1 severe case of anorexia nervosa per 200 schoolgirls and, for girls over age 16 in private schools, 1 case per 100. The incidence in the two state-run schools was much lower, approximating 1 per 550 students.

Subsequently a number of questionnaire surveys in this country and Western Europe have been conducted to study the prevalence (not incidence) of eating disorders. Depending on the definition of what constitutes a case, the prevalence of anorexia nervosa in women is between 0.7% and 2.1%, while that of bulimia is between 2% and 19% (see Table 3.2). Using stricter criteria for the latter disorder, most studies found that between 2% and 4.5% of the young women surveyed had a bulimic disorder. While the findings are quite consistent, the limitations of a questionnaire survey are considerable, primarily because the specificity and sensitivity of the questionnaires are unknown. Further, because of the low prevalence of the eating disorders in the general population, even a survey using an instrument such as the Eating Attitudes Test (EAT; Garner & Garfinkel, 1979) will still encounter the problem of the instrument's low positive predictive value (Button & Whitehouse, 1981; Williams, Hand, & Tarnopolsky, 1982); that is, most subjects with an EAT score above the threshold are in fact not cases of anorexia nervosa. Finally, the meaning of a high score on a certain questionnaire may be different for different populations (Eisler & Szmukler, 1985; Williams et al., 1982). Thus, for instance, Eisler and Szmukler (1985) found that the proportion of state-school girls having a high EAT score (7%) was actually greater than that of private-school girls (5%), although fewer of the former than the latter are actually cases of anorexia nervosa on direct interview.

At present the most widely accepted strategy is the two-stage screening survey (Williams, Tarnopolsky, & Hand, 1980), several of which for the eating disorders have been published (Table 3.3). The first stage involves screening a large number of individuals for probable cases by using a questionnaire, and the second stage involves trained researchers' interviewing such probable "cases" and usually also a number of randomly selected nonprobable cases in order to confirm their "caseness." To summarize their findings, the prevalence of anorexia nervosa is between 0.2% and 0.8%, and it is higher among the upper social classes. For private school girls aged 16 and over, the prevalence amounted to 1.1%, a figure comparable to that in Crisp and colleagues' (1976) study. The low prevalence of bulimia nervosa in Szmukler's (1983) study is puzzling. It suggests that bulimia nervosa perhaps has a later age of onset than anorexia nervosa; certainly

TABLE 3.2. Questionnaire Studies of the Prevalence of Eating Disorders

Study	Area	Population	AN	BN
Cooper & Fairburn (1983)	Southern England	369 F attending family planning clinic 14–40 yr	—	2% Russell's criteria
Halmi et al. (1981)	State University of New York	355 college seniors 33% M 60% F 14–67 yr	—	19% F *DSM-III* 5% M *DSM-III*
Healy et al. (1985)	Dublin College	701 F 361 M 17–25 yr	—	10.8% F *DSM-III* 1.1% M *DSM-III* 2.8% F and 0% M weekly episodes
Johnson et al. (1983)	Midwest high school	1,268 F 13–19 yr	—	8% *DSM-III* 4.9% *DSM-III* and weekly bingeing
Katzman et al. (1984)	Southwest college	485 F 327 M Psychology studies	—	3.9% *DSM-III*

Study	Setting	Sample		
Morgan & Sylvester (1977)	Bristol University	728 F 18 yr First-year students	2.1% history of AN	—
Nylander (1971)	Swedish high school	1,241 F 1,129 M 14–19 yr	*Girls* 0.7% definite cases 10% AN-like syndrome *Boys* None definite 1% AN-like syndrome	
Pope et al. (1984)	Suburban Boston	300 F over 12	0.7% *DSM-III*	10.3% *DSM-III* 3% *DSM-III* and weekly episodes
Pyle et al. (1983)	Midwest state universities	1,355 freshman	—	4.5% *DSM-III* and 0.4% weekly episodes

TABLE 3.3. Two-Stage Survey of Eating Disorders

Study	Location	Subjects	Method		Findings	
			1st stage	2nd stage	1st stage	2nd stage
Button & Whitehouse (1981), Whitehouse & Button (1988)	Southern England College of Technology	446 F 132 M Age = 16 to 22+ years	EAT	Interviewed 32 high scorers and 32 non-high scorers	32 F high scorers	0.2% AN (Feighner) 1.6% BN (DSM-III) 5% probably sub-clinical AN 3% "vomiters & purgers"; more common in Social Classes I & II
Clarke & Palmer (1983)	Leicester University	156 F 120 M 1st & 2nd year students	EAT CCEI	61% high scorers, 43% of borderline scorers inter-viewed	18 high EAT 7 borderline scorers, all F	No diagnosable AN 3% probable BN

Patton (1988b)	London comprehensive schools	1,010 F	EAT GHQ	Interviewed all high EAT scorers 2 control groups, all low EAT: (1) High GHQ (2) Low GHQ	Details not reported	0.17% AN + BN initially 0.26% AN + BN at 1-year follow-up (see text)
Szmukler (1983), Eisler & Szmukler, (1985)	London girls' schools	*Private school* 1,331 F Age 14–19 yr *State school* 1,676 F	EAT plus questions on weight, eating behavior, menses	Interviewed all high scorers and a sample of low scorers	5% private-school & 7% state-school high scorers	*Private school* 0.8% AN 0.4% BN 4% partial AN 1.1% AN in girls 16 and over *State school* 0.2% AN

clinical experience suggests that it often develops within the context of anorexia nervosa (Crisp, Hsu, Harding, & Hartshorn, 1980). All four studies found a substantial number of subclinical cases, but unfortunately the characteristics of these cases were not always clearly described. These subjects had symptoms suggestive of an eating disorder, although the symptoms did not meet the researchers' severity criteria to qualify as a case.

Finally, two groups of investigators, using questionnaires, have specifically studied the change in prevalence of bulimia nervosa in the same geographical area and in similar populations. Pyle, Halvorson, Neuman, and Mitchell (1986), in studying 1,389 freshmen in two midwestern universities, found the prevalence among female students who had probable bulimia nervosa to be three times higher in 1983 than 1980. However, Cooper, Charnock, and Taylor (1987) found no change in the prevalence among women attending a family planning clinic in the greater Oxford area in England in 1986 as compared to 1981 (Cooper & Fairburn, 1983). No obvious explanation exists for the discrepancy in these findings, unless, as we shall discuss in Chapter 4, the proportions of women dieting in these two populations were different. In any case, because these studies relied only on questionnaires, the findings are questionable. Whitehouse and Button (1988) reanalyzed their 1981 data (Button & Whitehouse, 1981) and found a prevalence of bulimia nervosa similar to that in Cooper's studies (Cooper & Fairburn, 1983; Cooper et al., 1987). However, since the investigators did not conduct a second survey, their finding could not be taken to indicate that there was no increase in the prevalence of bulimia nervosa.

EATING DISORDERS AMONG NON-CAUCASIANS

The prevalence of eating disorders among non-Caucasians in Western societies is not known. Several reports of the disorders in blacks have recently been published (for a review, see Hsu, 1987) and suggest that perhaps the disorders are affecting more blacks in this country and elsewhere. In non-Western cultures, relatively large series of both anorexia nervosa and bulimia nervosa have been reported in Japan (Nogami & Yabana, 1977; Suematsu, Ishikawa, Kubocki, & Ito, 1985), but the prevalence of the illnesses in that country is not known. In Malaysia, Buhrich (1981) contacted all psychiatrists and asked them to recall the number of cases of anorexia nervosa they had seen. Among approximately 60,000 new referrals over a period of 6 months to 26 years these psychiatrists could recall only 30 cases of anorexia nervosa, 28 females and 2 males. Over 90% of the patients were Chinese or Indian, although these ethnic groups constitute less than 50% of the population in Malaysia. Most of the patients were from higher social-class backgrounds. There was no apparent increase in the incidence of the disorder in Malaysia. In summary, the eating disorders do occur among non-Caucasian and non-Western cultures. They demonstrate the same clinical features and outcome, as well as the same female preponderance and tendency to occur among the upper socioeconomic classes.

In a survey of some 550 high school girls aged 14 to 16 in the Bradford (northern England) area, Mumford and Whitehouse (1988) found a higher prevalence of bulimia nervosa among the Asian (Indian and Pakistani) students than the Caucasian students (3.4% vs. 0.6%). However, it was unclear how acculturated the Asian students were. If replicated, this finding should confirm the primary importance of sociocultural influences on the pathogenesis of eating disorders.

HIGH-RISK STUDIES

Although the debate continues as to whether simple dieting is related to the onset of an eating disorder, clinical impressions suggest that an environment that emphasizes dieting and weight control may be conducive to the development of an eating disorder. Several studies that are focused on such at-risk populations have been published, with varying degrees of methodological sophistication, and have shed some light on the possible causative factors.

Druss and Silverman (1979), in a questionnaire study of 31 ballet students in New York, found the majority to show anorexia nervosa–like attitudes and behaviors. Garner and Garfinkel (1980) used a two-stage method to study 183 professional dance (mean age, 18.6 years) and 56 modeling (mean age, 21.4 years) students. On the EAT, 38% of the dance group and 34% of the modeling group had a high score, as compared to 9% of a mixed group of university and music students. On interviewing the high scorers and a sample of low scorers, 12 (6.5%) dance students and 4 (7%) modeling students but no university or music students were identified as having anorexia nervosa according to Feighner's criteria (Feighner et al., 1972). The majority of the individuals developed the illness while in the course of their studies.

More recently, Garner, Garfinkel, Rockert, and Olmsted (1987) assessed 55 11- to 14-year-old female students enrolled in a highly competitive, professional ballet school in North America, using only self-report questionnaires, including the Eating Disorder Inventory (EDI). Thirty-five of these students were followed up 2 years later by personal interview (including three not assessed initially). Fourteen were found to have an eating disorder: 9 had anorexia nervosa, 1 bulimia nervosa, and 4 a partial syndrome of either. In addition, 2 of the 23 students, who were not followed up because they had left the school, had definite anorexia nervosa. A high initial score on either the Drive for Thinness or Body Dissatisfaction scales of the EDI predicted subsequent diagnosable eating disorder; unfortunately it was unclear how many of the students already had an eating disorder at initial assessment. However, the high prevalence (over 25%) of eating disorders in this population lends support to the authors' original contention (Garner & Garfinkel, 1980) that pressures to be slim and successful contribute to the development of an eating disorder.

Yates, Leehy, and Shisslak (1983) interviewed approximately 60 marathon or trail runners and reported 3 male runners with anorectic-like symptoms. However, a subsequent study of marathon runners (Blumenthal, O'Toole, & Chang, 1984) found no definite cases of anorexia nervosa. Studies based on self-reports have found a high prevalence (25% or more) of pathological weight-control behaviors such as self-induced vomiting and use of laxatives or diuretics among male wrestlers (Enns, Drewnowski, & Grinker, 1987), female swimmers (Dummer, Rosen, Heusner, Roberts, & Counsilman, 1987), and female gymnasts (Rosen & Hough, 1988).

Two British studies have provided some direct support that dieting behavior, subclinical eating disorder, and diagnosable eating disorder occur on a behavioral continuum of severity and that the eating disorders are more prevalent when dieting behavior is common. Szmukler and colleagues (1985), in a study of 100 adolescent female ballet students in London, found seven (7%) to have diagnosable anorexia nervosa, while another three were borderline cases because their weight was higher than the researchers' strict criterion. All these individuals apparently developed their eating disorders during the course of their studies. Furthermore, significant eating disturbances were common among the other students: 37% had a fear of fatness, although they were actually below normal weight; 20% had previously lost a significant amount of weight, although, again, the amount of weight loss did not meet the researchers' strict diagnostic criterion and therefore these individuals were not diagnosable as having borderline or definite cases. This study clearly indicates that cases of dieting behavior, fear of fatness, weight loss, borderline cases, and diagnosable cases occur on a severity spectrum and that the prevalence of anorexia nervosa is higher when dieting behavior is common. Johnson-Sabine and colleagues (1988; Patton, 1988b), in a survey of 1,010 teenage girls attending eight London comprehensive schools, also found a spectrum of eating disturbances to exist among the schoolgirls, ranging from the feeling of being too fat to the syndrome of anorexia or bulimia nervosa. Furthermore, 21% of the dieters (defined by a high score on the EAT) on follow-up 1 year later had developed a diagnosable eating disorder, in contrast to only 3% of the nondieters. Higher weight, social difficulties, introversion, and family psychiatric history predicted the onset of an eating disorder at follow-up. Somewhat surprisingly, abnormal eating attitudes and the development of an eating disorder were apparently not related to social class. Unfortunately, these authors did not report in greater detail the subclinical cases, since they were grouped together with the definite cases, and figures for anorexia nervosa and bulimia nervosa were not reported separately. Nevertheless, this study again demonstrates that eating disturbances occur on a behavioral continuum and, because of its prospective design, provides direct evidence to suggest that dieting behavior, in the presence of other psychiatric and personality factors, may lead directly to the onset of an eating disorder.

Taken together, these studies suggest that an environment that emphasizes slimness and competitiveness leads to an increase in the incidence of the eating disorders as well as the prevalence of dieting behavior. Furthermore, they demonstrate that dieting behavior and diagnosable eating disorders occur on a behavioral continuum. Finally, they suggest that dieting may lead directly to the onset of an eating disorder for some individuals.

DIETING AMONG THE GENERAL POPULATION

This section reviews studies on dieting behavior in the general population, while Chapter 4 reviews those on attitudes toward shape and fatness.

Research has amply confirmed the popular impression that dieting is common among Caucasian women in the general population. Unfortunately, different studies defined dieting in different ways and thus the findings across studies may not be comparable. Furthermore, since many studies used only a questionnaire as the survey instrument, it is impossible to know whether the respondents understood the term *dieting* in the same way. Nevertheless, the findings converge and support the impression that many women consciously restrict their intake to control or lose weight and that the same factors that characterize eating-disorder patients also characterize dieting women.

Huenemann, Shapiro, Hampton, and Mitchell (1966) gave questionnaires each year to about 900 California high school students and traced their progress from the 9th through the 12th grade. The students' body fatness was also measured each year. Among the girls, 25% were classified as overweight by actual measurement, but more than 50% described themselves as fat and were concerned about it. Further, while the percentage of overweight girls remained quite constant throughout the 4 years, the number of girls who felt fat increased as they grew older. However, somewhat unexpectedly, the number of girls actually dieting to lose weight decreased from the 9th through the 12th grade. Caucasians and Orientals were much more likely than blacks to think themselves fat. In contrast to the girls, more than 50% of the boys felt they were too thin, and they seldom reported dieting. The number of boys who felt fat was somewhat less than those who were actually overweight. Twice as many black as Caucasian boys felt they were too thin. Almost all the boys wanted to be taller. Nylander (1971), in a questionnaire survey of more than 2,000 teenage boys and girls in Sweden, found similar results: The number of girls who reported feeling fat increased with age (28% of 14-year-olds and

50% of 18-year-olds), as did the number of those who were dieting (10% and 40% of 14- and 18-year-olds, respectively). Boys seldom reported dieting. Jakobovits, Halstead, Kelley, Roe, and Young (1977), in a questionnaire and food record survey of 195 Cornell University female juniors and seniors, found 11% to be on a diet and another 64% to be making a "conscious effort to limit the quantity" of food intake in order to lose or maintain weight (p. 408). Hsu, Milliones, Friedman, Holder, & Klepper (1982) surveyed 2,184 high school students in three northeastern urban and suburban districts, finding that 42% of the females and 17% of the males often felt fat and that 26% of the females and 8% of the males were dieting to control weight. However, according to the students' own reported weight, only 17% of males and 12% of females were actually overweight. Significantly, more white than black females were high scorers on the EAT. Johnson, Lewis, Love, Lewis, and Studkey (1983) surveyed 1,268 teenage schoolgirls in an urban high school. According to the researchers' definition of *dieting* as "an actual change of eating behavior for the purpose of losing weight," 36% were currently dieting and 69% had dieted in the past.

Further evidence that Caucasian women diet to control their fatness comes from a ten-state nutrition study (Garn & Clark, 1975, 1976). The study was conducted from 1968 through 1970 in ten states (Massachusetts, New York, Michigan, Kentucky, West Virginia, South Carolina, Louisiana, Texas, California, and Washington) to investigate the prevalence of both undernutrition and overnutrition. More than 40,000 subjects, both blacks and whites of all age categories, were studied. The findings that are relevant to our discussion include:

1. At all ages and among both blacks and whites, females tend to be fatter (as measured by triceps fatfold) than males.
2. Females tend to gain fat and males to lose fat during adolescence.
3. Among white females there is an income-related reversal of fatness during adolescence; that is, adolescent females in higher-income families start out being fatter but end up being leaner than those in lower-income families.
4. There is a reversal of fatness during adolescence of white and black females; that is, the former start out being fatter but end up being leaner than the latter during adolescence.

While there is no direct evidence to suggest that dieting actually results in slimness, the researchers had no doubt that the differential fatness patterns of black and white females and of higher- and lower-income white females were best explained by conscious dieting on the part of the white, higher-income adolescent females.

There is also some evidence to suggest that dieting behavior and more serious eating disturbances are related to the level of acculturation to Western ideals in a multicultural society. Hooper and Garner (1986) gave the Eating Disorder Inventory (EDI; Garner, Olmsted, & Polivy, 1983) to black, white, and mixed-race schoolgirls in Harare, Zimbabwe. A total of 399 girls around the ages of 16 to 18 responded. About 20% of them were high EDI scorers (on or above the 90th percentile for EDI score of North American college students); of these, 12.5% were black, 17.5% were of mixed race, and 70% were white. On interviewing an unspecified proportion of these high EDI scorers, the researchers found that anorectic and bulimic eating behaviors were most common among the whites and least common among the blacks, with the mixed-race group occupying an intermediate position. If confirmed, these findings would lend further support to the importance of sociocultural influences in the development of abnormal eating attitudes and behaviors.

DOES DIETING CAUSE THE ONSET
OF AN EATING DISORDER?

My contention is that eating disturbances ranging from simple dieting to subclinical to diagnosable eating disorders occur on a behavioral continuum. If this is the case, the prevalence of diagnosable eating disorders in a given population should be directly proportional to the prevalence of dieting behavior in the same population. The available evidence certainly supports this contention and suggests that dieting provides the entrée into an eating disorder. Nevertheless, not everyone who embarks on a diet will develop an eating disorder. Therefore other moderating influences must occur to precipitate an eating disorder. These factors are reviewed in Chapter 4.

4

Etiology

It is obvious to clinicians who have treated large numbers of eating-disorder patients that there is not a single event or factor that precipitates an eating disorder. Many researchers are therefore content to describe the etiology of the eating disorders as "multifactorial." However, the disorders affect quite selectively a certain sector of the population: those who are female, young, Caucasian, of upper socioeconomic status, and in a competitive environment that emphasizes slimness. Furthermore, the disorders seem to be increasing in prevalence in developed countries, and they apparently also affect Third World immigrants who have become Westernized. Any theory purporting to explain the etiology of the eating disorders must explain these findings. It would be difficult to imagine, for instance, that a primary hypothalamic disorder could manifest itself selectively only in such populations unless there are other intervening variables.

I hypothesize that dieting (i.e., a conscious restriction of food intake for whatever reason) provides the entrée into an eating disorder. Factors that intensify the dieting behavior therefore indirectly increase the risk of developing an eating disorder. Stated differently, eating disturbances ranging from simple dieting to diagnosable eating disorders occur on a behavioral continuum; the evidence for this has come from epidemiological findings that have already been reviewed (see Chapter 3). However, since the majority of those who embark on a diet do *not* develop an eating disorder, I further hypothesize that genetic, psychological, biological, personality, and family factors may increase the vulnerability of a dieting individual to an eating disorder. This chapter reviews the evidence for each of these factors.

SOCIOCULTURAL FACTORS

As discussed in Chapter 3, the prevalence of eating disorders in a given population seems to be directly proportional to the prevalence of dieting behavior in the same population. At present, dieting to control or lose weight is apparently prompted by two social trends in the West: an increase of fatness among the population and a desire to be thin.

There is some evidence to suggest that young men and women in the West are getting fatter. Recent average-weight statistics from the Society of Actuaries (1979) indicate that between 1959 and 1979 men in all age categories and women below the age of 30 became heavier, although the average weight of women over age 30 decreased. However, average-weight statistics may be misleading, since the increase in mean weight may simply be related to an increase in the prevalence of severe obesity while median weight remains unchanged. A study in Denmark (Christensen, Sonne-Holm, & Sorensen, 1981; Sonne-Holm & Sorensen, 1977) found that the prevalence of extreme obesity in young men in Copenhagen remained steady between 1943 and 1960 but increased sevenfold in the subsequent 14-year period. In young men in the provincial area of Denmark there was a fourfold increase in extreme obesity between 1964 and 1974. Both in and outside Copenhagen, the median body mass index of the young male population was unchanged.

The most likely explanation for the increase in fatness among the population of the West may be the abundance of food and the decrease in infectious diseases. Population studies among adults in India (Driver & Driver, 1983), Native American adults (Garb, Garb, & Stunkard, 1975), and children in Hong Kong (Chang, Lee, & Low, 1963) and the Philippines (Stunkard, 1977) have all demonstrated that increasing body weight is associated with an increased standard of living. This influence of social class on body weight is, however, reversed in the West. Goldblatt, Moore, and Stunkard (1965) studied 1,660 adults (690 males, 970 females) in midtown Manhattan and found obesity to be correlated with lower socioeconomic status: 30% of women of lower socioeconomic status were obese compared with 16% of middle-status and 5% of upper-status women. In addition, obesity was related to lower socioeconomic status of the individual's family of origin, downward social mobility, shorter duration of the family's stay in this country, and ethnic variables. The association of increased body weight with lower socioeconomic status in the West has been confirmed by studies in London (Baird, Silverstone, & Grimshaw, 1974; Silverstone, Gordon, & Stunkard, 1969); England, Wales, and Scotland (Braddon, Rodgers, Wadsworth, & Davies, 1986); southern Sweden (Hallstrom & Noppa, 1981); and Iowa (Halmi, Struss, & Goldberg, 1978). While there is no direct evidence to indicate that the slimness of those in the upper social classes is related to dieting, there is evidence to indicate that a desire to be slim is dependent on socioeconomic status. Dornbusch and colleagues (1984) studied a representative national sample of 7,514 youths between the ages of 12 and 17 with respect to this issue. After controlling for actual fatness, which was measured during a physical examination, adolescent females at every level of fatness in the higher social classes, whether measured by family income or by parental education, wanted to be thinner more often than those in lower social classes. In contrast, among adolescent males there was little relationship between social class and the desire to be thin.

The importance of being thin to middle- and upper-class women has been amply documented (Calden, Lundy, & Schlater, 1959; Jourard & Secord, 1955; Roden, Silberstein, & Stiegel-Moore, 1985; Singer & Lamb, 1966). For instance, Fallon and Rosen (1985) studied 248 male and 227 female undergraduates by using a set of nine figure drawings, ranging from very thin to very heavy. The students were asked to rate their current figure, their ideal figure, and the figure they felt would be most attractive to the opposite sex. For men, the current, ideal and most attractive figures were about identical. For women, the current figure was heavier than the most attractive, which in turn was heavier than the ideal. There is some evidence that this emphasis on slimness among women may be intensifying. By the time children are 7 or 8 years of age their concepts about physical attractiveness and slimness are very similar to those of older adolescents (Cavior & Dokecki, 1973; Cavior & Lombardi, 1973). In London, even 12- to 13-year-old girls expressed significant concerns about being too fat (Wardle & Beales, 1986). In reviewing weight and height data from *Playboy* centerfolds and Miss America contestants between 1959 and 1978, Garner, Garfinkel, Schwartz, and Thompson (1980) found a significant trend toward a thinner standard: In terms of average weight for height, there was about a 10% decrease over the 20-year period among these two populations. Meanwhile, they also found a sixfold increase in the number of diet articles in six popular women's magazines during the same 20-year period.

Cultural factors are also involved in prompting this desire for slimness. Chapter 3 reviewed studies showing that concern about fatness seems to be largely confined to young white females and that in Third World countries the severity of this concern seems to occur on a cultural continuum. Among Kenyan immigrants to Britain, Furnham and Alibhai (1983) found that traditional Kenyan women tended to rate larger female figures more favorably than Caucasian British women, while Kenyan British women who had been in Britain for at least 4 years were more similar to British women than to their Kenyan non-British counterparts in their perceptions. Furthermore, the study found that the British women's preference for small body shapes to the point of being anorectic was not uncommon. In this country, Pumariega (1986), in a study of 138 adolescent Hispanic females, aged 16 to 18, found a significant correlation between a subject's eating attitudes as measured by the Eating Attitudes Test (EAT; Garner & Garfinkel, 1979) and the level of her acculturation to American culture. Finally, in a pilot study of social attitudes toward anorexia nervosa, Branch and Eurman (1980) found that the friends and relatives of anorectics actually admired their control and slenderness.

In summary, the findings indicate that unless there is a conscious effort to limit dietary intake, increasing affluence is associated with higher body weight. Furthermore, the emphasis on slimness, a sociocultural phenomenon prevalent among upper-class females of the West, may be a major precipitant for the onset of an eating disorder. Nevertheless, not everyone who embarks on a diet will develop an eating disorder. Precipitation of an eating disorder by dieting must therefore be moderated by other factors. In view of the fact that the eating disorders occur most commonly during adolescence and among females, I hypothesize that adolescent turmoil, the development of self-concept and body concept, and identity formation in females are three issues that intensify this dieting process, which in turn may increase the risk of developing an eating disorder.

ADOLESCENT TURMOIL

The fact that the eating disorders occur almost invariably during adolescence suggests that developmental issues may be important in their pathogenesis. The idea that adolescence is a period of storm and stress was perhaps first popularized by Granville Stanley Hall, one of the major figures in the early history of American psychology. In an 1891 article he stated that adolescence is a period characterized by "lack of emotional steadiness, violent impulses, unreasonable conduct. . . . The previous self-hood is broken up . . . and a new individual is in the process of being born. All is solvent, plastic, peculiarly susceptible to external influences" (p. 207). This idea of adolescent crisis was taken further by many psychoanalysts. Anna Freud (1958), for instance, stated that adolescent emotional upheavals are inevitable, since they are the outward manifestations of the renewed battle between the ego and the id, with the former struggling for its very survival. She wrote: "Adolescence constitutes by definition an interruption of peaceful growth which resembles in appearance a variety of other emotional upsets and structural upheavals" (p. 267). And she further elaborates:

> I take it that it is normal for an adolescent to behave for a considerable length of time in an inconsistent and unpredictable manner; to fight its impulses and accept them; to ward them off successfully and to be overrun by them; to love his parents and to hate them; to revolt against them and to be dependent on them . . . to be more idealistic, artistic, generous and unselfish than he will ever be again, but also the opposite: self-centered, egoistic, calculating. Such fluctuations between extreme opposites would be deemed highly abnormal at any other time of life. (p. 275)

Blos (1970) echoed this view: "The more or less orderly course of development during latency is thrown into disarray with a child's entry into adolescence . . . adolescence cannot take its normal course without regression" (p. 11). In short, the psychoanalytic view asserts that a peaceful adolescence is in fact unhealthy and that neurotic or psychotic symptoms are often "normal" manifestations of such an upheaval, necessary and beneficial to growth. Again, to quote Anna Freud: "The adolescent manifestations come close to symptom formation of the neurotic, psychotic, or dissocial order and merge almost imperceptibly into borderline states . . . or fully fledged forms of almost all the mental illnesses" (p. 267).

However, recent research only partially supports such views. It is not true that adolescent crisis is inevitable; there are other pathways of growth (Offer & Offer, 1975). It is also untrue that psychiatric disorders are more benign in adolescence; the clinical picture of and prognosis for adolescent psychiatric disorders resemble very closely their counterparts in adults (Graham & Rutter, 1985). However, it is true that many adolescents, perhaps one out of two, are miserable (Kandel & Davies, 1982; Rutter, Cox, Tupling, Berger, & Yule, 1975), although such inner misery is generally unknown to others and does not seem to affect the youngsters' academic performance. Although it is also true that psychiatric disorders may be more common during adolescence than during childhood and adulthood (Rutter, Graham, Chadwick, & Yule, 1976), the majority of adolescents, perhaps three out of four, have no diagnosable psychiatric disorder.

How might adolescent turmoil cause an eating disorder? A striking finding in Western societies is that adolescent girls are more miserable than adolescent boys. Girls experience more anxiety, insecurity, and self-consciousness than boys (Bush, Simmons, Hutchinson, & Blyth, 1977–1978; O'Mally & Bachman, 1979; Savin-Williams, 1979; Tobin-Richards, Boxer, & Petersen, 1983), and this is particularly true for the white female adolescent (Simmons & Rosenberg, 1975). That this pattern may be cross-cultural is suggested by a study (Lerner, Iwawaki, Chihara, & Sovrell, 1980) that found Japanese female adolescents also to have lower self-esteem than their male counterparts. This unhappiness in the adolescent female may amount to significant depression. Kandel and Davies (1982) studied some 8,200 13- to 18-year-old students and 61% of their parents in upstate New York using the SCL-90 (Derogatis, Lipman, & Covi, 1973). They found that girls aged 14 to 18 had higher depression scores than their male counterparts and that this sex difference in depression was greater among the adolescents than among the parents. Furthermore, the generational difference between the depression scores of child and parent was greater for females than for males. Thus this study found that the female adolescent was the most depressed, followed in turn by the mother, the male adolescent, and the father.

This unhappiness of the adolescent Caucasian female is very likely a risk factor for the development of an eating disorder, since it may drive her to seek specialness and attractiveness through dieting and weight control. Kaplan, Busner, and Pollack (1988), in a study of 344 junior and senior high school students, found females who were underweight to be less depressed than those who were normal or overweight. In an earlier study, Kaplan, Nussbaum, Skomorowsky, Shenker, and Ramsey (1980) found that girls who perceived themselves to be overweight but were actually thin were more depressed than those who did not perceive themselves as fat. Noles, Cash, and Winstead (1985) found depressed subjects, both male and female, to be less satisfied with their own body sizes and shapes, although they were not rated as less attractive by a group of independent observers. In a British study of 50 non-eating-disordered female students aged 18 to 24, Taylor and Cooper (1986) found a significant correlation between depressed mood and overestimation of the subject's own body size. Finally, we have already mentioned Patton's findings (Patton, 1988b; see Chapter 3) that depression in high school students was significantly correlated with abnormal eating attitudes and behavior and that social difficulties and introversion, characteristics that may reflect increased adolescent turmoil, predicted the development of an eating disorder at 1-year follow-up.

SELF-CONCEPT AND BODY CONCEPT IN ADOLESCENCE

Research has repeatedly demonstrated that (1) there is a significant correlation between self-esteem, or self-concept, and satisfaction with body characteristics, or physical attractiveness and (2) this relationship is stronger for the female than for the male (Gray, 1977; Lerner & Karabenick, 1974; Tobin-Richards et al., 1983). Furthermore, in women more than in men, physical attractiveness is related to how an individual is evaluated by her peers, the quality of her peer relationships, and her personal prestige (Lerner, 1969; Staffieri, 1967). The cultural ideal of physical attractiveness is acquired early in the preschool years (Styczynsi & Langlois, 1977); as already mentioned, by the time children are 7 or 8 years of age, their concepts about physical attractiveness are very similar to those of older adolescents (Cavior & Dokecki, 1973; Cavior & Lombardi, 1973). Physical attractiveness in the female has been found to be the only important determinant of whether a man likes his date, at least among college freshmen (Walster, Aronson, Abrahams, & Rottman, 1966). Needless to say, therefore, physical maturation carries for the female many and varied connotations. While early maturation generally has a positive effect on the male adolescent and confers on him a greater sense of confidence and attractiveness, the effect of early maturation on girls is confusing and ambiguous (Jones & Mussen, 1958; Simmons, Blyth & McKinney, 1983; Tobin-Richards et al., 1983). On the one hand, it may give her greater popularity with the opposite sex; on the other, it may decrease her self-image and school performance. Hill and Holmbeck (1987), in a questionnaire study of 100 families of 7th-grade girls, found that the girls reported that, from the time of their menarche, they had experienced less acceptance from both parents, more parental control, and more disengagement on the part of the fathers. While this was an exploratory study, the findings are consistent with the popular view that sexual maturity in girls is a concern rather than a joy to the parents (Brooks-Gunn & Matthews, 1979). In the study by Dornbusch and colleagues (1984) we mentioned earlier, adolescent females who were sexually more mature (irrespective of chronological age) wanted to be thinner more often than those at an earlier stage of sexual maturation. In contrast, no such association occurred among the males. Thus it seems that physical maturation in the female carries more explicitly sexual meanings, which she and her family may find difficult to deal with.

Crisp (1967, 1980) has repeatedly suggested that anorexia nervosa reflects a phobic avoidance of sexual maturation and serves to protect the individual from adolescent turmoil; he has further suggested that the disorder tends to appear in families in which buried but unresolved parental conflicts would likely have been rekindled if the illness had not developed. I believe that the unsettling effects of sexual maturation at puberty may at least drive the female adolescent to a pursuit of thinness, which, she thinks, will bring her greater acceptance, self-control, and self-esteem. The finding that many 12- and 13-year-old London school-girls express significant concerns about their fatness and embark on diets (Wardle & Beales, 1986) supports this contention.

IDENTITY FORMATION IN THE FEMALE

There is also some evidence to suggest that the process of forming an identity may be particularly difficult for the female adolescent. The term *ego identity* was introduced by Erik Erikson (1955) to describe "both the persistent sameness within oneself (self-sameness) and a persistent sharing of some kind of essential character with others" (p. 57). While acknowledging that the term is vague and ambiguous, he nevertheless further elaborated its meaning as "a conscious sense of individual identity . . . an unconscious striving for a continuity of personal character . . . a criterion for the silent doings of ego synthesis . . . a maintenance of an inner solidarity with a group's ideals and identity" (p. 57). It is perhaps in regard to the last point that the female adolescent encounters the greatest difficulty, since the current societal ideal of a female is conflicting and confusing. It has already been mentioned that, in terms of physical attractiveness, the current ideal of feminine beauty is the lean, lithe look; that is, the young adolescent, early pubertal look (Faust, 1983). Since adolescent girls are more socially oriented than boys in their personality development, in that they rely more on social experiences and appraisals to define their self-concept (Carlson, 1963), such an unrealistic ideal of the female shape may be very disturbing. In his survey of 1,010 London high school girls, Patton (1988b) found that social difficulties and introversion, characteristics we take to indicate poor identity formation, were associated with the subsequent development of eating disturbances at 1-year follow-up. In a comparison of weight-preoccupied women and anorectic patients, Garner and colleagues (1984) found that some weight-preoccupied women were similar to anorectic patients in terms of a pervasive sense of ineffectiveness, a strong interpersonal distrust, and a lack of interoceptive awareness, characteristics we also take to indicate poor identity formation. Simmons and Rosenberg (1975), in a 1968 study of more than 1,800 boys and girls between 8 and 15 years of age in Baltimore, found adolescent girls, when compared to their male counterparts, to be more unhappy about being of their sex and less confident about their educational and thus presumably occupational opportunities in the future. Girls often define achievement in terms of their success in attracting the opposite sex and thus care much more than boys about how good-looking they are. This is particularly true for the adolescent white girl. Earlier, Douvan and Adelson (1966) also found girls to have more tentative and fuzzier perceptions of their future. However, such uncertainty about career choices may be changing. A more recent study (Konopka, 1976) found that most girls are planning to combine professional careers with motherhood. Nevertheless, girls aspiring to achieve dual careers may face other difficulties. Horner (1968) found that fear of success is much more prevalent in women than in men, and Hoffman (1974) suggests that a fear of loss of femininity and of interpersonal rejection may accompany success in a female. Orlofsky (1978) confirmed that fear of success in women is related to interpersonal rejection and loss of femininity and is highest in women who have already achieved an identity or are still striving to achieve one. Other researchers have confirmed that a female fear of success is more prevalent among those who are ambitious and nontraditional in terms of achievement and sex-role attitudes (Caballero, Giles, & Sharer, 1975; Heilbrun, Kleemeier, & Piccola, 1974). Thus it would appear that the feminist movement has so far brought mixed blessings for women.

Crisp (1967, 1980) has long held the view that anorexia nervosa is an avoidance of adolescent identity (particularly sexuality) undertaken in a society in which the female role is fuzzy and conflicting:

> I believe that such present widespread attempts of normal weight adolescent girls to reduce their fatness is a profound statement concerning the present nature of our society and the problem it has concerning restraint and impulse control. Such dieting, consciously aimed at promoting attractiveness, in the event fosters powerful internal control mechanisms necessary to many developing adolescents, who enter a society bereft of structure or much in the way of agreed behavior guidelines and codes of conduct. This social uncertainty is coupled with present day society's questioning of the inevitability of biological destiny, especially that of the female while at the same time inviting her to become "liberated." (1980, p. 52)

Meanwhile Bruch (1985), in asserting that anorexia nervosa is distinctly different from normal weight control, stated:

> My own observations suggest that the changing status of (and expectations for) women plays a role. Girls whose early upbringing has prepared them to become "clinging-vine" wives suddenly are expected at adolescence to prove themselves as women of achievement. This seems to create severe personal self-doubt and basic uncertainty. In their submissive way, they "chose" the fashionable dictum to be slim as a way of proving themselves as deserving respect. (p. 9)

Palazzoli (1978), while a maintainer of the primary role of the family in the pathogenesis of anorexia nervosa, nevertheless commented:

> Today . . . women are expected to be beautiful, smart and well-groomed, and to devote a great deal of time to their personal appearance even while competing in business and the professions. They must have a career and yet be romantic, tender and sweet, and in marriage play the part of the ideal wife cum mistress and cum mother who puts away her hard-earned diplomas to wash nappies and perform other menial chores. It is quite obvious that the conflict between so many irreconcilable demands on her time, in a world where the male spirit of competition and productivity reigns supreme, exposes the modern woman to a terrible social ordeal. (p. 35)

Orbach (1985) stated that all women are prohibited from expressing their own dependency needs or initiating social interactions, while at the same time they are encouraged to be deferential and "helpless" but caring, particularly in the arena of food preparation and feeding. Such conflicting demands, along with the dual image of the female body as sex symbol and as commodity, breed in the female adolescent feelings of insecurity and alienation toward her changing body. The striving for a "correct" body thus becomes a fundamental adolescent task.

It is my view, therefore, that the pathogenesis of an eating disorder is mediated by dieting to control or lose weight and that the factors that intensify this dieting indirectly increase the risk of developing an eating disorder. However, since most dieters do not proceed to develop an eating disorder, there must be other factors that moderate this process. There is evidence to indicate that genetic, psychodynamic, biological (mainly neurochemical), and family factors may play an etiological role. The evidence for these factors is reviewed below.

GENETIC FACTORS

Until recently, hereditary factors in anorexia nervosa had only been the subject of peripheral interest to investigators. Rainer (1982) has summarized the strategies that have been found to be most effective in research on the genetics of schizophrenia. These include: (1) analysis of pedigrees; (2) family-risk studies to determine the expectancy of the disorder in the relatives of patients as compared with the expectancy in the general population; (3) twin studies to determine the concordance rate of the illness in monozygotic and dizygotic twins; (4) adoption studies to tease out genetic and environmental influences by determining the rate of illness in patients' offspring adopted early in life by nonrelatives as compared with that in adoptees born to healthy parents; (5) high-risk studies to determine the development of psychopathology through observation of subjects with ill parents from childhood to adulthood; and (6) genetic marker studies to determine, for instance, whether certain enzyme activities are different between patients and healthy controls.

Systematic efforts to determine the genetic component in the eating disorders have occurred only in two of these areas: family-risk studies and twin studies. The findings of family-risk studies, reviewed in Chapter 2, unanimously demonstrate an increased risk for patients' relatives to develop an eating disorder. The earlier twin studies have been reviewed by Garfinkel and Garner (1982), Hsu, Holder, Hindmarsh, & Phelps (1984), and Nowlin (1983). Taken together, the studies reviewed by these authors involved 34 pairs of twins, but the zygosity of one pair and the concordance of a second were unknown. Garfinkel and Garner (1982) added information on nine pairs of their own and Nowlin (1983) on one pair. Thus among the 42 pairs with reported concordance and zygosity, the concordance rate for monozygotic twins was 47% (15/32) and for dizygotic twins, 10% (1/10). Several criticisms may be leveled against some of these early studies, such as doubtful zygosity, inadequate diagnostic criteria, and insufficient duration of follow-up of the nonanorectic twin. More recently, Holland, Hall, Murray, Russell, and Crisp (1984), in a collaborative study by St. George's and Maudsley hospitals in London, identified 34 pairs of twins and one set of triplets in which the probands had anorexia nervosa. The zygosity and diagnosis of the twins and triplets were all carefully confirmed. Of the 30 female twin pairs, 56% (9/16) of the monozygotic and 7% (1/14) of the dizygotic pairs were concordant for anorexia nervosa, while none of the male co-twins were concordant. It is also noteworthy that in the three male/female dizygotic pairs, it was always the female twin who had anorexia nervosa. Unfortunately, Holland and colleagues (1984) did not report on the proportion of restrictors versus bulimics in the probands or on whether the co-twins had subclinical forms of the eating disorders.

If the 13 pairs of twins from these studies with established zygosity (by blood-group analysis and/or placenta examination and resemblance of physical appearance) and explicitly stated diagnostic criteria (Table 4.1) are added to the St. George's and Maudsley series, the concordance rate for female monozygotic twins is 50% (14/28)

TABLE 4.1. Twins with Established Diagnosis and Zygosity

Number	Author	Zygosity	Concordance	Sex
1, 2	Askevold & Heiberg (1979)	MZ	D	F
3	Crisp (1965)[a]	MZ	D	F
4	Foster & Kupfer (1975)	MZ	D	F
5	Gifford et al. (1970)	MZ	D	F
6	Halmi & Brodland (1973)	MZ	D	F
7	Hsu et al (1984)	MZ	D	F
8	Mormont & Demoulin (1971)	MZ	D	F
9	Moskovitz et al. (1982)	MZ	C	F
10	Neki et al. (1977)	MZ	C	F
11	Nowlin (1983)	MZ[b]	C	F
12	Simmons & Kessler (1979)	MZ	C	F
13	Weiner (1976)	MZ	D	M

[a]Later included in Holland et al. (1984).
[b]Placental examination, all other pairs by blood-group analysis.

TABLE 4.2.   Combined Female Twin Data in Anorexia Nervosa

	MZ	DZ
Concordant	14 (50%)	1 (7%)
Discordant	14	13
Total	28	14

and for female dizygotic twins, 7% (1/14) (Table 4.2). The concordance for the two pairs of male monozygotic twins and one set of male triplets is 0%.

Reviewing the data for the discordant monozygotic pairs, Holland and colleagues (1984) could find no consistent difference between the pairs in terms of birth order, birthweight or educational success. Perinatal problems and childhood neurotic traits appeared to be more common for the anorectic twin, who also tended to be heavier in childhood, to be later to reach menarche (a somewhat unexpected finding in relation to earlier reviews on sex-role and sexual development), and to be less dominant. Hsu and colleagues (1984), in reviewing the data for eight pairs of monozygotic twins reported by other researchers to be discordant for anorexia nervosa, found the anorectic twin more likely to be the second born, the lighter at birth, and the more passive and submissive. Their own report of a pair of monozygotic twins concordant for bipolar disorder but discordant for anorexia nervosa indicated the anorectic twin to be less outgoing and more socially inept.

I am aware of no published twin studies for bulimia nervosa. In my own clinic, I have identified eleven sets of twins; eight pairs were female and three, male/female (see Table 4.3; Hsu, Chesler, & Santhouse, in press). Zygosity was established in all cases by the Physical Resemblance Questionnaire (Cohen, Dibble, Grawe, & Pollin, 1973, 1975) and in one case also by blood-group analysis. All patients fulfilled the DSM-III-R criteria for bulimia nervosa, and all were of normal weight. The concordance rate for the monozygotic twins (all females) was 33% (2/6) and for the dizygotic female (two sets) and male/female (three sets) twins, 0%. Family history of affective disorder and alcohol abuse was common (for further details on family

TABLE 4.3. Western Psychiatric Institute and Clinic Twins with Bulimia
Nervosa

	Female MZ	Female DZ	Female/male DZ	Total
Concordant	2	0	0	2
Discordant	4	2	3[a]	9
Total	6	2	3	11

[a]Patient was male in one set of twins; see text.

history see Table 4.4). However, the data must be considered preliminary.

The much greater concordance rate in the monozygotic twins
for anorexia nervosa and perhaps also for bulimia nervosa suggests the
presence of either a genetic predisposition or an environmental induc-
tion process in the pathogenesis of an eating disorder (Holland et al.,
1984). While the former explanation is more plausible, the latter can
only be ruled out by adoption studies and identification of genetic
markers. The importance of environmental factors is highlighted by
the case report of Crisp and Toms (1972) of an anorectic male whose
adoptive son and a girl who resided briefly with the family both
developed anorexia nervosa. If a genetic vulnerability is established, it
will then be necessary to identify how it predisposes an individual to
develop an eating disorder. A variety of possibilities exist, ranging
from a predisposition to poor affect and impulse control to an underlying neurotransmitter dysfunction. For anorexia nervosa, there is no
evidence to suggest more precisely what the mechanism might be. For
bulimia nervosa, I have speculated elsewhere (Hsu et al., in press) that
the genetic predisposition may be specifically related to affective
instability and poor impulse control, and that these characteristics in
turn predispose an individual to binge-eat when she embarks on a
strict diet. Finally, it is important to state emphatically that a genetic
vulnerability does not necessarily condemn an individual to developing an eating disorder. Even inborn errors of metabolism, such as
phenylketonuria, can be successfully treated with nutritional (i.e.,
environmental) manipulation. However, it would appear that an individual with a positive family history for an eating disorder is at greater
risk for developing one herself if she embarks on a rigid diet.

TABLE 4.4. Diagnosis in Probands, Co-Twins and Family

Proband[a]	Co-Twin[a]	Family[a]
1. Bulimia nervosa, major depression single episode, (diabetes mellitus)	MZ = no diagnosis	Sister = (seizure disorder) Brother = (brain tumor)
2. Bulimia nervosa	MZ = bulimia nervosa	Father = major depression recurrent and alcohol abuse Paternal grandmother = alcohol abuse, died of cirrhosis of the liver
3. Bulimia nervosa	MZ = no diagnosis	Sister = eating disorder not otherwise specified, alcohol abuse (obesity) Father = alcohol abuse
4. Bulimia nervosa, (obesity), (gastroplasty)	MZ = bulimia nervosa	Mother = (obesity, diabetes mellitus) Brother = (obesity) Brother = alcohol abuse (obesity)
5. Bulimia nervosa, major depression recurrent, alcohol abuse, mixed substance abuse, borderline personality disorder	DZ = major depression, alcohol abuse, mixed substance abuse, borderline personality disorder	Father = mother's third husband; alcohol and substance abuse; suicide at age 52 Mother = alcohol abuse; ? borderline personality disorder; twins brought up by foster parents from age 7
6. Bulimia nervosa	DZ = (obesity), (breast reduction surgery)	Both twins adopted away; biological family history unknown; adoptive mother (obesity), adoptive maternal grandmother = recurrent depression and suicide attempt, adoptive paternal grandparents = alcohol abuse.

92

Proband[a]	Co-twin	Family history
7. Bulimia Nervosa, past history of anorexia nervosa, (spina bifida)[b]	Female DZ = no diagnosis	No diagnosis
8. Bulimia nervosa, major depression recurrent, alcohol abuse, borderline personality disorder	Male DZ = no diagnosis	Sister = alcohol abuse Paternal uncle = major depression recurrent
9. Bulimia nervosa, major depression recurrent, alcohol abuse	Male DZ = alcohol abuse	Father = alcohol abuse Mother = (obesity), (diabetes mellitus) Maternal aunt = (obesity)
10. Bulimia nervosa, major depression, single episode, in remission	MZ = no diagnosis	Paternal aunt = suicide
11. Bulimia nervosa	MZ = dysthmia	Father = died of leukemia at 43; alcohol abuse

[a]Axis III diagnosis in parenthesis.
[b]Male proband.

INDIVIDUAL PSYCHOPATHOLOGY,
PERSONALITY, AND PSYCHODYNAMICS

The evidence we have reviewed thus far suggests that an individual who embarks on a diet is more likely to develop an eating disorder if she is experiencing significant adolescent turmoil, has a low self-concept and body concept, and is having difficulty with identity formation. Stated differently, psychiatric co-morbidity (such as depression and social anxiety) in an individual may precipitate an eating disorder if she is dieting. Some evidence to support this contention has been supplied by Patton (1988b), who found that social difficulties and introversion were associated with the subsequent development of eating-disorder symptomatology. Furthermore, outcome studies of both anorectic (e.g., Cantwell et al., 1977) and bulimic (e.g., Hsu & Sobkiewicz, in press-b) patients have found depression, social phobia and anxiety, and obsessive–compulsive features to be prominent in some patients at follow-up. It is impossible at this stage to decide whether these concurrent symptoms are primary or secondary to the eating disorder, and much more research needs to be conducted to clarify the role of co-morbidity in the pathogenesis of an eating disorder.

We have already reviewed the personality findings for eating-disorder patients (see Chapter 2). Some researchers (e.g., Strober, 1981) hold the view that the core personality disturbances of these patients may be central to the pathogenesis of an eating disorder. For the anorectic, affective overcontrol and intolerance, lack of self-direction and personal effectiveness, and relative absence of adaptive functioning to the maturational tasks of adolescence have been identified as possible causal factors; while for the bulimic, affective instability and poor impulse control are considered to be important.

Obviously, we may use languages derived from other conceptual frameworks to describe these findings. Historically, etiological theories focused on the individual have been predominantly psychodynamic in nature. As early as 1931, Brown postulated that anorexia nervosa was a pathological manifestation of the detachment of the growing individual from parental authority. He further stated that a fear of growing up and anxiety about responsibility were highly characteristic of anorectic patients. Bruch (1973, 1982) has repeatedly asserted that anorexia nervosa is the individual's attempt, on the one hand, to gain competence and respect by being slimmer and, on the other, to ward off feelings of helplessness, ineffectiveness, and power-lessness by imposing severe discipline on her own body. The anorectic disorder is thus related to underlying deficits of self, identity, and autonomy. She further postulated that such deficits occur because the parents have superimposed their own wishes on the child without paying attention to her expressions of needs and wants. The would-be patient is therefore unusually good, successful, and gratifying as a child; but when faced with the demands of adolescence, she becomes aware of an inner emptiness and powerlessness. Because of her pre-conceptual and concrete thinking, the result of not being allowed to develop independence in thought and feeling, she seizes on society's glorification of thinness and turns weight loss into a struggle for a sense of identity, purpose, specialness, and control. Attempts to test the many aspects of Bruch's ideas have begun only recently. Garner and colleagues (1984) have found that anorectic women, when com-pared with weight-preoccupied women, have a greater sense of inef-fectiveness and interpersonal distrust, as well as a greater lack of interoceptive awareness. However, Bruch's idea of body-image distur-bance remains unproven despite much research, and the parent–child interaction pattern is apparently more pathological for the bulimic anorectic than for the restrictive anorectic (Humphrey, 1987; Strober et al., 1982).

Crisp (1967, 1980) has also repeatedly stated his view on the pathogenesis of anorexia nervosa. He has emphasized that puberty is triggered upon reaching a threshold weight, which the anorectic is seeking to avoid. He therefore believes that the anorectic displays a phobia of adolescent weight, not a fear of fatness. Since this threshold weight is associated with biological maturity and sexuality, its attain-ment brings with it major implications for both the individual and the family. Adolescence is thus a period during which the individual has to come to terms with her genital sexuality; to integrate it into her ways of relating to her peers, both male and female; to differentiate herself from her family; and to renegotiate her relationship with her parents. Crisp has postulated that the would-be patient and her family are unable to deal with such a maturational crisis, and anorexia nervosa is thus an adaptive stance a patient has taken to avoid first the pubertal weight and secondarily its maturational consequences. In Crisp's view anorexia nervosa is thus a weight-based phobic avoidance posture. Support for Crisp's view has come indirectly from two areas: Frisch and her colleagues (Frisch & McArthur, 1974; Frisch, Wyshak, & Vincent, 1980) have shown that menarche and menstruation in a female hinges on the individual's obtaining a critical amount (approximately 25% of body weight) of fatness, and Boyar et al. (1974) have found that the immature pattern of gonadotropin release in anorectic patients reverts to normal after weight gain. Whether the patients have an actual weight phobia is, however, difficult to substantiate (Salkind, Fincham, & Silverstone, 1980), since self-starvation serves not only to avoid a phobic stimulus but also to pursue the gratifying goal of thinness.

Early psychoanalytic theories based on a drive-conflict model postulated that anorectic self-starvation is a defense against fantasies of oral impregnation (Waller, Kaufman, & Deutsch, 1940) or oral sadistic cannibalism (Masserman, 1941) or both (Grimshaw, 1959). However, apart from the fact that such fantasies are not common in anorexia nervosa, these postulations do not adequately explain the characteristic fear of fatness or the sense of inward emptiness. Later, object-relations theories postulated that there is an underlying deficit in the anorectic's development of object relations, particularly during the oral incorporative stage. Palazzoli (1978) considered that the anorectic has equated her body with her maternal introject, a bad, overcontrolling object that she has incorporated and identified with. Self-starvation is therefore an attempt to terminate this identification within her body and to strive for a sense of separate identity. Sours (1980) has also described the anorectic self-defects in terms of poor self–object differentiation and failure to develop self and object constancy. By their very nature such concepts are difficult to prove or disprove. However, oral incorporative fantasies and identification of their bodies with their mothers are clinically uncommon among anorectics (Goodsitt, 1985). Selvini Palazzoli has since seemingly abandoned an object relations view for a family oriented one. Recently, analysts have written about the etiology of anorexia nervosa from a self-psychology perspective (Goodsitt, 1983, 1985). It is postulated that in normal development, maternal functions, such as soothing, stimulation, and protection, become transferred to a transitional object (such as a blanket), which the child controls and which in turn provides her with a sense of well-being and security. The child recognizes the transitional object as something external but experiences it as a part of herself. With "good enough" mothering, the child internalizes these functions and they become part of her mental structure. It is further postulated that in the eating disorders this internalization process is aborted as a result of disturbance in the mother–child relationship. The deficit in self-structure is liable to make the individual feel ineffective, out of control, empty, and unworthy. Life is passively experienced. This view thus converges with those of Bruch (1973, 1985), but again it is difficult to verify. Borderline personality disorder, which shares many of the features described, occurs in 10% (Pope et al., 1987) to 50% (Levin & Hyler, 1986) of bulimics, and its occurrence rate in anorectics is likely to be lower.

The cognitive–behavioral theory of the etiology of anorexia nervosa emphasizes the proximal cognitions and behaviors that cause and maintain the disorder. Garner and Bemis (1982, 1985) and Garfinkel and Garner (1982) postulate that the various causal factors finally converge at one point: the patient's belief that "it is absolutely essential that I be thin." Dieting thus occurs to avoid the feared stimulus of fatness and its implications, such as psychosocial maturity. Such avoidant behavior is difficult to extinguish and may actually be perpetuated by the patient's increasing isolation, which decreases her responsiveness to other issues and considerations. Further, the anorectic behavior is maintained by the positive reinforcement of thinness, which provides a sense of gratification, self-control, and mastery, not to mention approval and concern from others. Finally, cognitive distortions and dysfunctional thoughts, such as dichotomous reasoning and catastrophizing, further maintain the illness behavior. For bulimia nervosa researchers have set forth a cognitive-behavioral theory based on a functional analysis of cognitions and behaviors involved in the binge-and-purge process (Fairburn, 1981; Rosen & Leitenberg, 1985; Slade, 1982). Antecedents for a binge include prolonged dieting leading to feelings of hunger and deprivation as well as such negative feeling states as dysphoria, a sense of failure, self-critical thoughts, anxiety, or frustration in relation to outside stress for which the subject has limited coping skills. Other investigators have emphasized the importance of restrained eating as an antecedent. Restrained eaters are found to increase their intake when made to feel anxious (Herman & Polivy, 1975), when distressed (Polivy & Herman, 1976), when consuming alcohol (Polivy & Herman, 1976), or after they believe they have broken their diet and thus failed

(Fremouw & Heyneman, 1984). Boskind-Lodahl and White (1978) hypothesize that the binge episodes provide the bulimic with a release from tensions and dilemmas and that such tensions and dilemmas are directly related to strivings to achieve an exaggerated ideal of femininity and acceptance from men. Food represents the only area of her life that a bulimic can indulge excessively without fear of disapproval or reprisal, at least for the moment.

Because the cognitive–behavioral model focused on the proximal causes and maintenance variables, it is compatible with other models of etiology (Garner & Bemis, 1982). Further, it makes intuitive sense and is consistent with patients' own descriptions of the illness process. However, by its very nature it does not explain why some dieters develop an eating disorder while others do not, or why some develop anorexia nervosa while others develop bulimia nervosa.

BIOLOGICAL THEORIES

Russell (1970, 1977a, 1985) has repeatedly stated that a disorder of hypothalamic function may play a role in the pathogenesis of anorexia nervosa. There exists overwhelming evidence for a hypothalamic disorder in anorexia nervosa and, to a lesser extent, bulimia nervosa, but such disturbances are almost always secondary to malnutrition and weight loss. Recent investigations have focused on central nervous system neurotransmitters (see Chapter 2). Rapid advances in the area are occurring and reviews of the findings rapidly become out of date. Currently no compelling evidence exists to suggest that there is a primary (i.e., not related to weight loss and/or malnutrition) central nervous system deficit in norepinephrine, serotonin, or opioid systems in anorexia nervosa or bulimia nervosa. However, the fact that starvation leads to binge-eating and the dramatic response sometimes encountered with bulimic patients given antidepressants or fenfluramine (see Chapter 6) suggest that research in the neurotransmitters is likely to yield fruitful results in the future.

THE ROLE OF THE FAMILY

Evidence has already been presented that unipolar and bipolar affective disorders, alcohol and substance abuse, and eating disorders are more prevalent among the first- and second-degree relatives of both anorectic and bulimic patients (Chapter 2). An individual with such a family history who goes on a diet may therefore be at greater risk for developing an eating disorder, although the mechanism whereby such a family history might precipitate an eating disorder is unclear. Perhaps the tendency for poor affect and impulse regulation renders the would-be patient more likely to use rigid dieting for control and binge-eating for comfort. Alternatively, perhaps a biological vulnerability, such as a deficiency of some neurotransmitters, is responsible.

For some time, however, investigators have focused on the role of dysfunctional family interactions in the pathogenesis of the eating disorders. Many early writers were aware of the pathological interaction between the anorectic patient and her family (see Chapter 2). For instance, Lasegue (1873) wrote that "both the patient and her family form a tightly knit whole, and we obtain a false picture of the disease if we limit our observations to the patients alone." The idea that the family is directly responsible, at least in part, for the pathogenesis of the eating disorders is, however, more recent. Many writers (e.g., Bruch, 1973, 1978; Crisp, 1980; Kalucy et al., 1977; Palazzoli, 1978; Sours, 1980) have described a typical anorexia nervosa family, aspects of which have been summarized by Yager (1982). In brief, the family is often portrayed as middle to upper class, successful, concerned about external appearances and physical fitness, anxious to maintain outward solidarity and harmony, and concerned to uphold rigid but usually unspoken family rules at the expense of open communication (and hence unable to resolve conflicts or express negative feelings, such as anger or jealousy). Members relate as if they could read one another's minds. The parents are said to be experience-denying, reluctant to assume personal leadership and responsibility, prone to blame their decisions on others and disinclined to acknowledge their personal preferences and needs. It is postulated that the would-be anorectic patient brought up in such a family will find it particularly difficult to deal with issues of separation and individualization, of achieving a personal identity, and of accepting her adult sexuality.

Most authors seem to suggest that such family issues are not specific to the condition of anorexia nervosa. Minuchin and his colleagues (Minuchin et al., 1975; Minuchin & Fishman, 1981), however, have suggested that certain transactional patterns are characteristic of psychosomatic families, those marked by anorexia nervosa included. *Enmeshment* refers to the high degree of involvement in such families—their excessive togetherness, intrusion on personal boundaries, lack of privacy, poorly differentiated perception of self and other family members, and weak family subsystem boundaries. Relaying of messages is common, and members often speak for each other, thus blocking direct communication. *Overprotectiveness* refers to the excessive nurturing and concern for one another's welfare. Somatization and pacifying behaviors are common. *Rigidity* refers to the family's heavy commitment to maintaining the status quo. Changes are threatening and dealt with by avoidance mechanisms. *Lack of conflict resolution* occurs because of the family's low conflict tolerance, frequent use of detouring mechanisms, and rigidity and overprotectiveness. These four transactional characteristics provide the context for the sick child to use her illness as a mode for communicating overtly avoided messages and a mechanism for avoiding family and parental conflict. For psychosomatic illnesses such as diabetes mellitus and bronchial asthma, Minuchin and his co-workers postulated a physiological vulnerability and seemed to suggest that the dysfunctional family transactional patterns acted to exacerbate the already present physiological symptoms. For anorexia nervosa, which they classified as a secondary psychosomatic disorder, they left open the question of a possible physiological vulnerability but seemed to suggest that emotional conflicts within the family system are transformed into somatic symptoms. They did not discuss the possible mechanism of such transformation. More recent writings from the group (Sargent, Liebman, & Silver, 1985) have apparently retreated from such claims and instead refer to the family characteristics as the "context in which the primary psychological features of anorexia nervosa . . . fit and are adaptive" (p. 260). Thus even this vociferous group now seems to regard the family more as an "enabler" than as a primary causative factor. The lack of well-controlled data to support these claims has already been reviewed in Chapter 2. One "follow-back" case report indicated that some abnormal mothering might have occurred during the childhood of a 28-year-old male anorectic (Rampling, 1980). Crisp and colleagues (1974), using a standardized measure, found that the psychoneurotic status of parents worsens significantly as they gain weight with treatment and that this is particularly so if the parental relationship is poor. Furthermore, they found 6-month outcome to be related to the initial level of parental psychopathology. These findings, however, are difficult to interpret: case selection factors, family therapy effects, and observer bias were not controlled for. Finally, we have already described the more recent efforts to study family interaction patterns by standardized methods (see Chapter 2, section on Family Characteristics). The findings all suggest that eating-disorder families have more disturbed interactions than normal families, but we lack evidence to indicate that such disturbances are the cause of the eating disorder. In summary, much more work needs to be done to clarify whether, in fact, anorectic families show a characteristic interaction pattern, whether the pattern is a necessary precondition for the pathogenesis of the disorder or occurs as a consequence of the illness, and whether dysfunctional transactions perpetuate the illness behavior.

TOWARD A COHERENT THEORY
OF ETIOLOGY

I have already stated my hypothesis that "normal" adolescent dieting provides the entrée into an eating disorder if such dieting is intensified by adolescent turmoil, low self and body concept, and poor identity formation. The risk is further increased if there is a family history of affective or eating disorders or alcohol or substance abuse. Other risk factors may include certain personality traits, such as long-standing feelings of emptiness and ineffectiveness, overcontrol of emotionality, conformity, and, in the case of bulimia nervosa, poor affect and impulse regulation. Significant psychiatric symptoms, such as depression, social anxiety and phobia, and obsessive–compulsive features, if they occur concurrently with the dieting behavior, may also precipitate an eating disorder. Genetic factors may operate through any of these factors.

The most common proximal reason for dieting nowadays is to control or lose weight to attain a thin body. Since the intensity of such behavior is related to being overweight, it is not surprising that being overweight has been found to predict the subsequent development of eating disturbances in adolescent girls (Patton, 1988b). Dieting may also occur in response to nonspecific stressors, such as family discord or moving to a new environment (see Chapter 2, section on Precipitating Events), since they are often equated with self-control and discipline, which are attributes needed to cope with the stress. In previous times dieting probably occurred mainly for religious reasons, which again were usually related to self-discipline or control. In accordance with our hypothesis, prolonged religious fasting could also lead to the development of pathological eating disturbances, and perhaps it is for this reason that the eating disorders were not entirely unknown in earlier times, although they were not recognized as such (Bell, 1985).

Once the pathological eating disturbances are established, they may then be perpetuated by both positive and negative reinforcers, the former including the exhilaration and triumph associated with the weight loss and the approval and attention of others, and the latter including the fear of fatness and its attendant meanings, such as psychosexual maturity. Willful starvation for whatever reason is always a powerful interpersonal statement and may be used to express anger or elicit concern. Family transactional dysfunction may serve both as a positive (e.g., because the illness increases a sense of solidarity) or negative (e.g., the illness leads to avoidance or detour of conflict) reinforcer. The cognitive and conceptual distortions also perpetuate the illness and may be related to a disturbance in self-structure or to a dysfunctional parent–child interaction. Early upbringing may influence any of the factors listed above, but evidence to support its direct etiological role is lacking. The evidence for a primary hypothalamic/neurotransmitter dysfunction, possibly triggered by the initial dieting, is inconclusive but may explain how the anorectic can sustain her prolonged willful starvation without giving in to the impulse to eat.

Bulimia clearly occurs as a result of semistarvation or restraint, suggesting a deranged compensatory mechanism, possibly mediated by hypothalamic/neurotransmitter dysfunction. In time it also serves to regulate affect and impulse, and thus the behavior self-perpetuates. Vomiting or purging usually occurs to avoid weight gain but may itself regulate affect and impulse; either way it serves to perpetuate the binge-and-purge behavior. Genetic predisposition, personality factors, family transactional patterns, and perhaps early upbringing experiences may determine whether a pathological dieter develops anorexia nervosa or bulimia nervosa.

Finally, in the pathogenesis of an eating disorder, I believe that genetic and environmental factors are not mutually exclusive. Genetic predisposition may, among other influences, affect personality development, which in turn affects the environment. The challenge is to identify how these factors operate to produce an eating disorder.

5

Evaluation and Diagnosis

The initial evaluation of an eating-disorder patient serves to establish a diagnosis, determine the severity of illness, detect any concomitant psychiatric or physical complications, and generate a treatment plan. In addition, continual assessment of the patient and family is necessary during treatment; this allows the clinician to understand their strengths and weaknesses, to formulate the factors that precipitated or perpetuate the illness, and to evaluate for treatment effect.

Cantwell and Baker (1989) have suggested that the diagnostic evaluation of any psychiatric disorder involves the following: (1) a diagnostic process of making inquiries about the patient, (2) a set of diagnostic tools for systematic data collection, (3) a diagnostic system to classify the disorders, and (4) an assimilative process to interpret the data and determine if they fit a particular diagnostic scheme.

In actual practice the diagnostic tools that one uses determine to a large extent the questions that one asks. The assimilative process essentially involves generating, from the data gathered, the diagnosis and differential diagnosis. In this chapter I describe my own evaluation process and discuss the various issues involved in the diagnosis of the eating disorders.

THE DIAGNOSTIC EVALUATION PROCESS

The initial diagnostic evaluation is usually completed in the first two sessions, each lasting about 2 hours. However, as will be discussed in Chapter 6, this process may take longer if much time and effort is spent in engaging the patient and family to become collaborators in treatment. This section should therefore be read in conjunction with the section on Engaging the Patient and Family as Collaborators in Chapter 6. In the initial consultation, when first meeting with the patient and the family, I ask the patient whether she would prefer being seen initially on her own or with the family. If the former, I interview her alone (the process is described in Chapter 6, section on Engaging the Patient and Family as Collaborators). If she prefers the latter or expresses no particular preference, as is the case for the majority of patients in my experience, then I usually begin by meeting with the patient and the family together to discuss each person's general impression of the presenting problem. In the brief joint interview, the clinician can sometimes gain an impression of the family's style of interaction, which may shape the subsequent conduct of the interview. For instance, if the mother does all the talking for the family, I may specifically solicit the father's views. At this stage, I am always encouraging and supportive, generally simply accepting each member's comments without confrontation. If the parents have many questions, I spend time addressing at least some of them. I also take this opportunity to discuss the issue of confidentiality; unless there is an urgent reason, I will not discuss with the parents what the patient has said in confidence. Other basic rules of treatment are discussed in the second session, when the treatment plan is presented. At this point I may inform the parents about the cost of the initial consultation, if this has not already been done.

Following this joint interview I spend about 1 hour with the patient to collect pertinent clinical information. Although the interview is conducted in a semistructured way, I always encourage the patient to say what she has on her mind rather than only to answer my questions.

Weight and Dietary History

The patient is always weighed in indoor clothing and without shoes, and her height taken at the first interview. How much the patient wants to weigh (i.e., ideal or desired weight) is often a good indication of how severe the weight phobia is and may lead to a discussion of how she feels about her body at different weights. I then ask for the maximum and minimum adult weight and any weight fluctuations. I try to determine the length of time the patient has maintained her weight at each level and whether weight fluctuations were associated with any significant life events or changes in dietary habits.

For a patient with anorexia nervosa, I then ask the patient to describe her eating pattern on a typical weekday, as well as on weekends. I try to speak the patient's language in the inquiry, as recommended by Orbach (1985). The first onset of dietary restriction is determined, as are the events surrounding it and her weight and menstrual pattern at the time. I ask for the results of the dieting, how much weight was lost in what period of time, and how she felt about it. The patient may volunteer information about binge-eating, and if she does not I usually probe with such questions as: "When people go on a diet to lose weight, they sometimes feel so hungry that they are tempted to eat a whole lot. Have you experienced that?" The patient's idea of a binge should be noted. Information about vomiting and other methods of purging, if not volunteered, are usually asked for in a roundabout way: "Have you tried to lose weight by any other means?" If the answer is no, I usually defer exploration until later. I then ask the patient to describe how she feels about her body and whether the feelings have changed with changes in weight.

For the bulimic patient, I also begin by asking for a description of her intake on a typical weekday, and on the weekends. I then ask for details of the binge episodes—their frequency, the most common times of occurrence, their duration, and the types and amounts of food eaten. She is also asked to describe her thoughts and feelings before, during, and after a binge. Some patients may feel very embarrassed, and repeated reassurance and explanation about the purpose of the inquiry may be necessary. Some patients may emphasize the negative feelings during a binge ("I feel awful but I don't know why I do it"), and it may be helpful to point out that during the first few minutes of a binge most, if not all, patients feel a sense of relief, satisfaction, nurturance, or oblivion. The patient may thereby begin to understand and accept that some of her binges do occur for a reason. Patients should also be asked to describe their thoughts and feelings before, during, and after vomiting or purging. All patients purge to get rid of the calories, some enjoy the fact that they can eat what they want without gaining weight, a few, usually those with concurrent borderline personality disorder, find the purging to have a relaxing or cleansing effect. Some patients spit their food out, but they seldom volunteer this information. I probe by asking whether she uses other ways to get rid of her food and calories. I then ask for her feelings about her body.

For both the anorectic and the bulimic patient, it is often helpful to get an idea of how she views her food, whether she divides it into good and bad categories and the reasons for doing so. Some understanding of who does the cooking and food shopping and how food is prepared or served may also be useful for treatment planning. Shoplifting is common for bulimics, but I usually defer inquiring into this area until later.

Alcohol and substance abuse are more common for bulimics, but I routinely ask about alcohol and drug use (including diet pills, diuretics, laxatives, and syrup of ipecac) with every patient. However, I sometimes defer this until the evaluation of the patient's mental state.

Menstrual and Sexual History

Menstrual pattern, periods of menstrual irregularity, amenorrhea, and the age of onset of menses should always be documented. The correlation of her menstrual period with body weight and eating behavior, as well as her affective state, should also be discussed with the patient. I ask her about feelings regarding menstruation and amenorrhea. I then ask for her thoughts and feelings about and her interest in sex and, in the older patient her actual sexual behavior. About 15% to 20% of bulimic patients I have evaluated in the last few years have described significant sexual trauma, either rape or incest, prior to the onset of their eating disorders.

Mental State

I ask specifically for symptoms of depression, such as feelings of sadness, low self-esteem, loss of interest and motivation, sleep disturbances, feelings of hopelessness, and suicidality. Although recognizing that many of these features may occur as a result of the eating disorder, I am less concerned about whether these symptoms are primary or secondary to the eating disorder. They should be documented if present and carefully monitored in treatment. I also ask for symptoms of anxiety states, including social anxiety and panic attacks, and for obsessive–compulsive and psychotic features. Self-injurious behavior, suicide attempts, and other impulsive features, including alcohol and substance abuse, are asked about. Personality characteristics and quality of interpersonal relationships are assessed at this point. Although I collect information in a systematic fashion, I do not normally use a standardized structured interview as a diagnostic tool unless the patient is entered in a research protocol.

Social and Developmental History

The developmental history is usually taken in the context of the history of the present illness. Any significant developmental problems or birth difficulties are recorded. Birthweight, childhood weight, and early feeding patterns are considered important by some investigators. I inquire about her social relationships outside the family by asking such questions as how many people comprise her circle of friends, whether she has a best friend, what she has in common with her friends, and what aspects of her peer relationships she would like to see changed. I ask her to describe her daily routine on weekdays, weekends, and vacation days and ask specifically about her participation in organized activities. I assess her academic achievement and goals by asking her about her current grade level, her best and worst subjects, and her future academic and career goals. I also ask for her perception of her family's expectations regarding her academic achievement and goals.

Previous Treatment

About 50% of patients who come to my clinic have had previous treatment elsewhere. I ask for their experience regarding this treatment and whether and how they have benefited from it. I ask about any medications she may have taken or is still taking and ask for consent to obtain the treatment records.

Family History

I specifically ask for the following information on each family member (grandparents, parents, and siblings), usually in the context of constructing a family tree: age, height, weight, occupation, state of physical health, history of eating disorders, affective illness, alcohol or substance abuse, and any other psychiatric or physical disorders. Significant psychiatric or physical history in the extended family is also recorded. Even if there is no family history of overt eating disorders, I ask about family attitudes regarding weight and eating. I also ask for each family member's reaction to the patient's illness. If any family member is deceased, I ask for the age and cause of death and for the patient's and family's reactions to the bereavement. Family relationships and alliances may be explored at this stage or left until later, depending on whether I feel that adequate rapport has been established.

I then ask the parents to join the patient to discuss their views about her illness. If the parents want to see me without the patient, I always ask their permission to discuss later with the patient the information they have given in her absence. Any gaps in the family history may be filled in at this point. I then give the patient and parents my general impression of the illness; schedule a second assessment session, which will include a physical examination; and answer any questions the patient and parents may have. In the context of answering their questions, I usually describe the effects of starvation, the various etiological factors in general, and the course and outcome of the illness. I also outline the principles of treatment and mention that more specific treatment recommendations will be made at the end of the second session. Again, I am supportive and encouraging, avoiding escalating conflicts and striving to join with the patient and family in a collaborative effort (Minuchin et al., 1978). If blame shifting or guilt-ridden comments arise, I make statements to the effect that it is always difficult to know whose fault it is for what and that the pathogenesis of the disorder is always complex. If a parent asks specifically what he or she can do to help the patient eat more or stop bingeing, I always refer the question to the patient by saying: "This is a very important question, why don't we ask what _____ thinks?" Commonly the patient will request that the parents back off, and at this stage I ask the parents to go along with the patient's wishes, at least for the next few weeks. I may then spend some time discussing with the patient what she can handle with her eating during the coming week before the next appointment. I emphasize the importance of eating small amounts of a balanced diet three times a day, not to gain or lose weight but simply to maintain her weight at presentation until the next appointment.

In the second session, I meet with the patient and the family to fill in any gaps in the data collection. The bulk of the second session is spent in taking a medical history and performing a physical examination.

Medical History and Physical Examination

Taking a medical history and performing a physical examination for an eating disorder patient are not different from doing these with other patients. In my experience about 5% of patients have a concurrent major medical illness, such as diabetes mellitus or epilepsy, in addition to the eating disorder. In my clinic a nurse practitioner usually performs the physical examination under the supervision of a physician. Medical complications have already been described in Chapter 2. The following laboratory tests are done on all our patients: complete blood count; electrolytes; creatinine, and blood urea nitrogen assessments; urine analysis, including microscopy; and an electrocardiogram. Other tests are ordered as necessary.

Standardized Interviews and Self-Report Measures

Each eating-disorder clinic probably has its own standard practice of data collection. Of the commonly used psychiatric interviews, the Diagnostic Interview Schedule for Children (Costello, Edelbrock, Dulcan, Kalas, & Klaric, 1980) and the Structured Clinical Interview according to *DSM-III-R* (SCID; Spitzer, Williams, Gibbon, & First, 1988) both contain a section on the eating disorders. The SCID has the additional advantage of being able to generate an Axis II diagnosis. Johnson (1985) has published a questionnaire, the Diagnostic Survey for Eating Disorders, which covers not only the eating disorders but also medical and psychiatric history, life adjustment, and family history. However, it has not been standardized. Self-rating scales and questionnaires may provide useful supplementary information. For the average clinician, I recommend the use of simple self-report measures, such as the Beck Depression Inventory (Beck, Ward, Mendelson, Mock, & Erbaugh, 1961) and the Eating Attitudes Test (Garner & Garfinkel, 1979). Such self-report measures are easy to score and serve as a useful guide for monitoring progress when they are given periodically during treatment.

Treatment Recommendations
and Periodic Review of Progress

At the end of the evaluation I recommend a treatment plan. I discuss the treatment setting, that is, inpatient versus outpatient, according to the indications described in Chapter 6. For outpatient treatment, I usually begin with individual and family therapy and discuss with the patient and family the focus and content of treatment and the purpose of each. I sometimes assign one therapist to do both treatments and sometimes assign separate therapists, depending on patient preference and staff time and availability. I have no particular preference for either approach, feeling that each has its merits and drawbacks. For instance, therapist splitting is easier to deal with when both patient and family see one therapist, but trust and confidentiality issues are sometimes problematic. Some patients find it comfortable to establish a boundary by having a personal therapist she does not share with the family. In my clinic, group psychotherapy is instituted only when some progress has been made in individual and family therapy. All outpatients are asked to make at least one appointment with a registered dietician, and for bulimic patients I am currently utilizing a detailed program of nutritional counseling, which will be described in Chapter 6. Medication is almost never started right away; it is usually given if indicated after a few weeks of observation. The rules governing confidentiality, sharing of information, appointment times, cancellation of appointments, contacting the therapist outside of appointment times, and cost of sessions are then discussed. Finally, I recommend that the patient and family attend a local support group.

It is essential that the patient's clinical condition be monitored and reviewed at regular intervals during treatment. Since the course of illness is usually lengthy for an eating disorder, the needs of the patient and the family may change over time. In the initial stages of treatment a patient may benefit from, say, a psychoeducational approach, whereas as she overcomes her eating difficulties she may benefit from a more psychodynamic type of treatment. If the condition of a patient has not improved after a reasonable period of time, the therapist should perhaps consider seeking a second opinion to discuss whether a change in treatment plan is necessary. Treatment plans and treatment goals must be reviewed periodically and revised if necessary.

THE PURPOSE OF MAKING A DIAGNOSIS

In the field of medicine the value of classifying and diagnosing diseases is generally unquestioned. Classification is the process whereby complex clinical phenomena are reduced to defined categories for the purpose of treatment and prevention, while diagnosis is the assignment of the patient's clinical features (e.g., constrictive chest pain occurring upon exertion in a 50-year-old man with exercise ECG changes and coronary atherosclerosis) to a particular category (e.g., angina pectoris) for the purpose of treatment (e.g., nitrates and beta-blockers) and secondary prevention (e.g., weight reduction). However, in psychiatry classification and diagnosis are often deemed irrelevant to the nature of the problem. Thus, for instance, a diagnosis of anorexia nervosa does not convey vital information, such as why the patient needs to strive for control, who brought her to treatment, or how she relates to her family. Furthermore, in other branches of medicine treatment is usually directly related to diagnosis, whereas in psychiatry specific treatments are rare. Thus classification and diagnosis are of less value for treatment planning in psychiatry. Finally, some psychiatrists feel that it is dehumanizing and harmful to fit a patient's symptoms into a classificatory scheme; they insist that a patient should be understood as an individual and treated as a person.

Why, then, are we concerned about classification and diagnostic criteria? Classification is based on the assumption that there are certain shared features among disorders that distinguish one particular category of disorder from all the others; a related assumption is that patients with this category of disorder can be distinguished from those without it. Classification is therefore essential for delineating and defining the condition that one proposes to treat. It is also essential for the purpose of communication with others, so that we can all know what particular mental disorder we are describing. A third reason is that it is essential for learning, for comparing with one another our experience of treating patients with the same disorder.

Finally, it is important for developing specific prevention and treatments. While these are still rare in psychiatry, it is nevertheless essential that we set the stage for the evaluation of such efforts by clearly defining the conditions.

However, to argue for the value of diagnosis in psychiatry is not to overlook its shortcomings. Thus, in clinical practice, the assignment of a diagnosis should always be accompanied by a detailed formulation of the patient's clinical features, personality features, personal and social history, family history and relationships, and previous treatments.

THE CATEGORICAL AND CONTINUOUS MODELS FOR DIAGNOSIS

If we take the position that simple dieting and the eating disorders occur on a behavioral continuum (see Chapters 3 and 4), where do we draw the line for distinguishing a "case" of an eating disorder from a "noncase?" In the remainder of this chapter it will become clear that I think operational criteria are necessary, at least at present, to define a case. Stated differently, I believe that a case is a case when certain characteristics in addition to the dieting behavior are present; for instance, features of emaciation and fear of fatness.

To adopt both a continuous and a categorical model is not to commit an act of obscurantism. In a discussion on the "caseness" of childhood depression, Eisenberg (1986) suggests that both models should be used simultaneously to increase our understanding of a particular disorder. Using the example of the relationship between height (a continuous model) and dwarfism (a categorical model), he suggests that extreme shortness in stature is associated with an increased probability of a variety of dwarfism, although it is not height per se that distinguishes the "pathologically" short from the "normally" short. Similarly, I argue that extreme dieting is associated with a case of an eating disorder, which is distinguishable from a noncase by the presence of certain clinical features. However, the dieting behavior itself is not what distinguishes a case of eating disorder from a noncase. Since I also believe that these associated features are not qualitatively different from similar (albeit less severe) ones present in "normal" dieters, I acknowledge that the line drawn to distinguish a case from a noncase on any given continuum is arbitrary. However, in psychiatry we are at the stage of defining disorders by clinical signs and symptoms. We are therefore governed by such questions as, "What cluster of signs and symptoms makes the most sense?" and "Where do I draw the line in terms of severity?" In the following section, I suggest that it is the constancy of association of the signs and symptoms, the severity of a particular sign or symptom, the uniformity of outcome, and the implications for treatment that should determine our definition of categories. Of course, as knowledge increases, our current definition of disorders will be replaced by one based on pathological and/or etiological classifications.

DIAGNOSTIC ISSUES AND SYSTEMS

The emergence of the eating disorders as diagnostic categories has been hampered by two major difficulties. The first is a lack of agreement on how diagnostic criteria should be established. The traditional approach to establishing diagnostic categories is to provide brief descriptions of the characterisic features of each condition. The problem related to this approach is the lack of precision that limits the usefulness of classificatory schemes thus defined. A more recent approach is to provide adequate working (i.e., operational) definitions of the various diagnostic categories; examples of this approach are the system of Feighner and colleagues (1972) and the American Psychiatric Association's *DSM-III* (1980) and *DSM-III-R* (1987) systems. The correct use of such operational criteria allows a clinician to make a fairly precise description of the patient sample.

A second hurdle is a lack of agreement and understanding among investigators as to the etiology, cardinal features, course, and outcome of the eating disorders. Chapter 1 has already described the historical development of the concepts of anorexia nervosa and bulimia nervosa. However, even recent investigators, such as Feighner and colleagues (1972) still considered the weight loss in anorexia nervosa to be due to anorexia (i.e., a loss of appetite), and many clinicians apparently still regard anorexia nervosa as an appetitive disorder. The distinction between anorexia nervosa and bulimia nervosa is still a subject of debate among researchers. However, with the establishment of the *DSM-III* and *DSM-III-R* criteria, at least we now have a point of departure for our discussion on the diagnostic issues.

Dally (1969) made one of the earliest attempts to provide operational diagnostic criteria for anorexia nervosa. As necessary conditions for the diagnosis of anorexia nervosa, he listed (1) a steadfast refusal to eat; (2) weight loss of at least 10% of previous weight; (3) amenorrhea of at least 3 months' duration; and (4) absence of schizophrenia, psychotic depression, or organic disease. This approach was extended by Feighner and colleagues (1972), who limited the age of onset to before age 25 and listed as necessary conditions (1) a weight loss of at least 25%; (2) a distorted and implacable attitude toward eating food or weight that overrides hunger, admonition, reassurance, and threats; (3) no known physical or other psychiatric disorder to account for food refusal or weight loss; and (4) at least two of six manifestations, which include amenorrhea, lanugo, bradycardia, periods of hyperactivity, bulimia, and vomiting.

A more conceptual approach was adopted by Russell (1970) and Crisp (1977). Russell stated his three criteria thus: (1) The patient's behavior leads to a marked loss of body weight and malnutrition, behavior that includes fasting, selective carbohydrate refusal, self-induced vomiting, purgative abuse, or excessive exercise; (2) there is an endocrine disorder that manifests itself clinically by amenorrhea in the female and loss of sexual interest and potency in the male; and (3) there are present a variety of mental attitudes, such as a morbid fear of becoming fat, a belief that to be thin is to be desirable, a loss of judgment regarding food intake and body weight, and sometimes depressive and phobic symptoms. Crisp (1977) stated that the diagnosis has to be made on three levels, the first being the observable clinical features of emaciation, loss of reproductive capacity, restlessness by day and insomnia by night, and such stigmata of starvation as a reduced metabolic rate, lanugo, and cyanotic peripheries. He further distinguished between the abstainer (i.e., restrictor) and the bulimic subgroups. The second level consists of the central psychopathological feature of anorexia nervosa; namely, the steadfast, overriding, often denied preoccupation with first pursuing a low body weight and then maintaining it within the context of an increasing phobia about biologically normal adolescent weight and attendant fatness. The third level is the psychosocial environment within which the disorder has developed, particularly that of the family; especially important here are the family's emphasis on such middle-class values as perfection, success, and fitness and its limited capacity to deal with the turmoil of adolescence. However, Crisp has emphasized that this third level is probably not specific to anorexia nervosa. These conceptual definitions are difficult to implement reliably in practice.

For bulimia nervosa Russell (1979) originally proposed two diagnostic criteria: (1) an irresistible urge to overeat, followed by self-induced vomiting or purging, and (2) a morbid fear of becoming fat. Later he refined and expanded on these criteria (Russell, 1985): (1) The patient is much preoccupied with thoughts about food and succumbs to episodic gorging; (2) she attempts to mitigate the fattening effects of food by one or more of the following—self-induced vomiting, purgative abuse, and alternating starvation, appetite suppressant drugs, or other devices with a similar aim; (3) the psychopathology of the disorder is a morbid fear of fatness, usually shown by the patient's setting herself a sharp weight threshold below her optimum, or "healthy," weight; and (4) she has experienced an earlier episode of anorexia nervosa, which may have been fully expressed or may merely have asssumed a cryptic form with a loss of weight and/or amenorrhea lasting a few months.

In his revised criteria, Russell again avoided giving numerical cutoffs, and his criteria are therefore difficult to apply consistently in practice. For instance, what constitutes a "cryptic" form of anorexia nervosa may easily vary from clinician to clinician. Furthermore, to include the bulimic form of anorexia nervosa in the diagnosis and to specify a history of anorexia nervosa create, in my view, unnecessary confusion. I will comment further on these issues later in this chapter.

The American Psychiatric Association (1980) took the operational approach and distinguished bulimia from anorexia nervosa. More recently the DSM-III-R (see Tables 5.1 and 5.2) has made several welcome changes in the criteria. For anorexia nervosa, it has specified the necessity of a low body weight, deleted the controversial term *disturbance in body image*, and added the criterion of amenorrhea for three consecutive cycles. For bulimia nervosa, it has distinguished the symptom of bulimia from the syndrome of bulimia nervosa; specified the frequency of binges; stipulated that the presence of vomiting, purging, and/or exercising is necessary for a diagnosis of the syndrome; and added a persistent concern with body shape and weight as a criterion.

TABLE 5.1.   DSM-III-R Diagnostic Criteria for Anorexia Nervosa

A.   Refusal to maintain body weight over a minimal normal weight for age and height, e.g., weight loss leading to maintenance of body weight 15% below that expected; or failure to make expected weight gain during period of growth, leading to body weight 15% below that expected.

B.   Intense fear of gaining weight or becoming fat, even though under-weight.

C.   Disturbance in the way in which one's body weight, size, or shape is experienced, e.g., the person claims to "feel fat" even when emaciated, believes that one area of the body is "too fat" even when obviously under-weight.

D.   In females, absence of at least three consecutive menstrual cycles when otherwise expected to occur (primary or secondary amenorrhea).

Note. From *Diagnostic and Statistical Manual of Mental Disorders* (3rd ed., rev.) (p. 67) by The American Psychiatric Association, 1987, Washington, DC: Author. Copyright 1987 by The American Psychiatric Association. Reprinted by permission.

TABLE 5.2.   DSM-III-R Diagnostic Criteria for Bulimia Nervosa

A.   Recurrent episodes of binge eating (rapid consumption of a large amount of food in a discrete period of time).

B.   A feeling of lack of control over eating behavior during the eating binges.

C.   The person regularly engages in either self-induced vomiting, use of laxatives or diuretics, strict dieting or fasting, or vigorous exercise in order to prevent weight gain.

D.   A minimum average of two binge eating episodes a week for at least three months.

E.   Persistent overconcern with body shape and weight.

Note. From *Diagnostic and Statistical Manual of Mental Disorders* (3rd ed., rev.) (pp. 68–69) by The American Psychiatric Association, 1987, Washington, DC: Author. Copyright 1987 by The American Psychiatric Association. Reprinted by permission.

Can the *DSM-III-R* Criteria Be Improved?

In commenting on the *DSM-III* criteria for anorexia nervosa, I have elsewhere (Hsu, 1986) suggested that both weight loss and low weight should be specified. (For a summary of recommended diagnostic criteria for anorexia nervosa, see Table 5.3.) Criterion A of the *DSM-III-R* now specifies both low weight and weight loss. However, it now gives only the cutoff for weight (15% below that expected) and has removed amount of weight loss as a criterion. This certainly simplifies the weight criterion, but it is unclear if this change is warranted. I still believe that severity of emaciation should be speci-

TABLE 5.3.   Proposed Diagnostic Criteria for Anorexia Nervosa

1. Intense fear of becoming obese or a relentless pursuit of thinness that does not diminish as weight loss progresses.
2. Behavior directed toward weight loss: self-imposed starvation, excessive exercising, and self-induced vomiting or purging.
3. Weight loss of at least 25% of original body weight.
4. Emaciation: Stage 1—body weight at 75% to 85% of average; Stage 2—body weight at or below 75% of average.
5. In the female: amenorrhea of at least 6 months' duration.

fied (i.e., Stage 1—15% to 25% below average; Stage 2—more than 25% below average). I support the inclusion of amenorrhea as a criterion (Criterion D) out of deference to tradition, although I acknowledge that it is still unclear if in fact the amenorrhea reflects a primary hypothalamic disorder and, if not, what precise significance it has (other than its occurrence as a phenomenon secondary to weight loss and starvation). I still favor a separation of anorexia nervosa into the restrictor and bulimic subgroups for reasons to be discussed below. I believe that a category for subclinical anorexia nervosa should be created instead of lumping it into Eating Disorders Not Otherwise Specified (NOS), and the reasons for this are also discussed below.

I believe that the diagnosis of bulimia nervosa should be confined to individuals of normal weight. (For a summary of recommended diagnostic criteria for bulimia nervosa, see Table 5.4.) There is some evidence to suggest that the outcomes of normal-weight bulimia nervosa and the bulimic form of anorexia nervosa are different (see Chapter 7). Furthermore, many bulimic anorectics binge or vomit only occasionally and thus would not meet the *DSM-III-R*'s frequency criterion (Criterion D). Are they to be diagnosed as having anorexia nervosa? If so, the distinction on the basis of frequency of episodes seems artificial. A diagnosis should carry some treatment implications, and the treatment of a normal-weight bulimic is quite different from that of a bulimic anorectic, which is much more similar to that of a restrictive anorectic. As already mentioned, Russell (1985) proposed that a history of overt or cryptic anorexia nervosa be a necessary criterion for the diagnosis of bulimia nervosa. I disagree with this view simply because there is no evidence to indicate that those with such a history have a different clinical picture or outcome

TABLE 5.4.   Proposed Diagnostic Criteria for Bulimia Nervosa

1. Recurrent episodes of binge-eating.
2. Recurrent episodes of self-induced vomiting or use of laxatives and/or diuretics to prevent weight gain.
3. A minimum of two binge-eating episodes a week for at least 3 months.
4. Persistent overconcern with body shape and weight.
5. Body weight within ± 15% of normal.

from those who do not (Hsu & Holder, 1986; Lacey, 1983). (For a comparison of the clinical features of anorexia nervosa and bulimia nervosa, see Table 5.5.) Finally, I believe that a category for subclinical bulimia nervosa should be delineated.

Eating Disorders NOS is now used as a category to include all eating disorders that do not meet the criteria for a specific eating disorder. This category is unsatisfactory, since it fails to delineate subclinical anorexia nervosa from subclinical bulimia nervosa and from other eating disorders. The outcomes of subclinical anorexia nervosa and subclinical bulimia nervosa deserve to be studied specifically so that we may understand the progression of symptoms and whether the disorders "breed true." I therefore suggest that subclinical anorexia nervosa and subclinical bulimia nervosa (based on the fact that neither meets the severity criteria of the respective disorder) be separated from Eating Disorders NOS, which can then be used as a category for other less well-defined disorders of eating.

TABLE 5.5.   Comparison of Clinical Features of Anorexia Nervosa and Bulimia Nervosa

| Features | Anorexia nervosa | | Bulimia nervosa |
	Restrictor subgroup	Bulimic subgroup	
Weight loss	Severe	Severe	Minimal to moderate
Body weight	Very low	Low	Normal
Amenorrhea	Present	Present	Variable
Bulimia	Absent	Present	Present
Vomiting/purging	Absent	Present	Present
Fear of fatness	Present	Present	Present

Differential Diagnosis

The differential diagnosis of anorexia nervosa consists of other conditions that produce weight loss. Medical conditions such as Crohn disease and psychiatric illnesses such as major depression may sometimes lead to diagnostic confusion. However, the cardinal feature of fear of fatness is always absent in these patients. Weight loss from other psychiatric disorders, such as schizophrenia, obsessive-compulsive disorder, or conversion disorder, may occur, but usually the clinical features of the primary disorder are prominent. Again, there is no fear of fatness for these patients. Comparing a group of 20 patients with a conversion disorder presenting with vomiting and weight loss and a group of 20 patients with anorexia nervosa, Garfinkel, Kaplan, Garner, and Darby (1983) found the two groups to differ significantly in terms of their preoccupation with weight, body size, and dieting.

Conversion disorder presenting with vomiting may also be confused with bulimia nervosa, but the fear of fatness and binge-eating will be absent. In my view, the correct diagnosis of bulimia nervosa is not usually difficult if the patient presents with specific eating problems. Difficulties arise, however, in two situations. The first is the underdetection of concurrent, secondary symptoms, whether or not they are related to the bulimia nervosa. Clinically, many bulimic patients also qualify for a secondary diagnosis of major depression, alcohol/substance abuse, or borderline personality disorder (see Chapter 2), but clinicians are sometimes so preoccupied with the eating disorder that the concurrent disorders are overlooked. The second difficulty occurs when the patient presents with a non-eating-disorder complaint. Many of my bulimic patients who have been treated for another psychiatric disorder have never told their psychiatrist about their bingeing-and-purging behavior. In a small series of five elderly eating-disorder patients, three had previously seen a psychiatrist for affective disorder but the eating disorder was not detected (Hsu & Zimmer, 1988). I therefore recommend that in the evaluation of a psychiatric patient the clinician routinely ask about the patient's dietary habits and weight history.

In summary, the purpose of the initial evaluation of a patient who has presented with an eating problem is to make a diagnosis and, if warranted, a list of differential diagnoses. Because the patient is almost always frightened and defensive the clinician should be supportive and active in the evaluation process. Much effort should be spent in engaging the patient and the family and in educating them regarding the illness and the treatment process.

CASE ILLUSTRATION

The following case is presented to describe the assessment process in my clinic and to illustrate the techniques I have used to engage the patient and family. I provide a brief commentary at the end and, in the next chapter, will use the same case to illustrate the treatment process. Needless to say, details of the case have been changed to prevent identification.

Pam—height, 5'6"; weight, 122 pounds—was a 17-year-old high school junior who came to the clinic with a 2-year history of bulimia, vomiting, and abuse of diet pills. Just over 2 years ago she had decided to go on the diet to lose a few pounds because the instructor at the charm school she was attending thought she was overweight at 125 pounds. Subsequently she enlisted with a modeling agency and her agent insisted that she get down to 110 pounds. In addition to putting herself on a 900-calorie diet, Pam began using over-the-counter diet pills, increased her exercising, and, when the desired amount of weight loss did not occur, swallowed air to self-induce vomiting after meals. Within a few weeks she brought her weight down to 110 pounds but then began bingeing. After bingeing and vomiting secretly for 18 months, she told her mother about it. Her father, who had been advised by his physician to stop smoking because of his angina pectoris, made a pact with Pam: If she stopped vomiting, he would stop smoking. This led to no apparent improvement over a 6-month period; by the time she came to the clinic, she was bingeing and vomiting up to three times a day and using up to eight diet pills per week.

Family history was positive for major depression in the paternal grandmother, for which she was hospitalized, and for alcoholism in the father, which was untreated. The patient was an only child; the father, who was 20 years older than the mother, had been married before. The parental relationship was strained, and during the parents' frequent arguments Pam was often pressured into declaring her loyalty to either one or the other of her parents.

The mother brought Pam to the initial assessment. The father did not come; he said he was busy and thought psychiatric treatment was not necessary for Pam. Both Pam and her mother were convinced that treatment was necessary but felt the father might stop them from coming to the clinic. The nurse conducting the intake interview telephoned the father to ask if he could come to the next appointment but he declined, giving no reason. The mother said he probably would not meet with the nurse because he "despises all women." The psychiatrist therefore called the father and, indeed, he agreed to attend a session with him alone. During this session, which occurred a week after the initial assessment, the father stated that he did not believe Pam needed any treatment but promised not to interfere with her sessions. He realized that Pam was concerned about his drinking but insisted that he had it under control. He admitted to problems in the marriage but did not feel any marital counseling would be of any benefit. He refused to attend any family sessions.

During the initial assessment the patient was given a number of questionnaires to complete in addition to the formal psychiatric interview. The results are summarized in Table 5.6.

On the Schedule for Schizophrenia and Affective Disorder (Endicott & Spitzer, 1978) Pam was found not to be suffering from a major depression. The Beck Depression Inventory (BDI; Beck et al., 1961) score of 12 (cutoff generally accepted to be around 20) was within the normal range, supporting the absence of clinical depression. The Eating Attitudes Test (EAT; Garner & Garfinkel, 1979) score was 29, which is high (cutoff about 20), and the Eating Disorders Inventory (EDI; Garner, Olmsted, & Polivy, 1983) score was 47, which is also high. The Symptom Checklist (SCL-90; Derogatis et al., 1973) score was 12, which is low and suggests an absence of severe overall psychopathology. Pam's Social Anxiety and Distress Scale (SAD; Watson & Friend, 1969) and Fear of Negative Evaluation (FNE; Watson & Friend, 1969) scores were higher than those of college-age (i.e., older) women, who have a mean SAD of about 8 and a mean FNE of about 16.

Comment

This case is not unusual in terms of its presentation and history. The assessment results are also in keeping with what one would expect to find in most young women with bulimia nervosa. The treatment team

TABLE 5.6.   Assessment Findings of Case Illustration

	At intake	After 8 weeks of treatment	After 1 year follow-up
Binges per week	10	0	0
Vomiting episodes per week	20	2	0
EAT	29	7	4
EDI	47	18	11
BDI	12	1	7
SAD	27	27	28
FNE	20	22	21
SCL = 90	12	3	11

felt it was important to meet with the father on at least one occasion to explain the treatment process and ensure that he would not interfere with treatment. He indeed kept his promise, and although family therapy was not possible, at least the patient and her mother were able to attend the sessions regularly. The treatment and outcome of this case will be described in Chapter 6.

6

Treatment

The eating disorders are intriguing illnesses that demonstrate the complex interaction among intrapsychic and interpersonal processes as well as biological and sociocultural factors. However, while the treatment of these young and intelligent patients is usually rewarding, the clinician must bear in mind that these are potentially life-threatening illnesses and some patients may become chronically ill.

It may be stated at outset that the treatment of the eating disorders is largely pragmatic and should be directed at the major areas of dysfunction (Halmi, 1983). Treatment goals should always be clearly formulated and treatment plans carefully and conscientiously implemented. The use of sound principles and good clinical judgment is crucial, since there are relatively few properly conducted treatment studies to guide the clinician. For anorexia nervosa, although there has been no major breakthrough in its treatment in the last 25 years, a number of issues have been clarified by recent research. Furthermore, we finally have some data to suggest that treatment may at least improve the short-term outcome of the disorder (see Chapter 7). For bulimia nervosa, there are several treatments of proven efficacy, at least in the short term. This chapter first discusses three general issues: the qualities needed in a therapist, the importance of engaging the patient and family as collaborators in treatment, and the breaking of confidentiality. For the sake of clarity, the treatments of anorexia nervosa and bulimia nervosa are discussed separately. Treatment studies are reviewed systematically, and when the findings conflict or expert opinions differ, recommendations are offered.

GENERAL ISSUES

Qualities of a Therapist

The treatment of an eating disorder necessarily involves an intense and usually prolonged interaction between therapist and patient. It is therefore difficult to imagine that the qualities of the therapist do not vitally affect the outcome of the encounter. However, very little has been written specifically on this topic. Crisp (1967, 1980; Crisp, Norton, Jurczak, Bowyer, & Duncan, 1985) has repeatedly stressed the importance of the staff's being able to control their own countertransference toward the patient; unfortunately he did not elaborate on it. Garner, Garfinkel, and Bemis (1982) and Strober and Yager (1985) emphasize the importance of a flexible style, a caring attitude, and a genuine concern in the therapist. They also emphasize that in order for the patient to develop a sense of trust, the therapist should be truthful about every detail of the proposed treatment. Finally, they also consider it important for therapists to be able to bear the feelings of hopelessness, manipulation, and powerlessness within patients as well as cope with the frustration and anger patients arouse in them; that is, be able to control their own countertransference. In addition, Strober and Yager (1985) provided a long list of attributes that they deem vital for a therapist working with an adolescent anorectic patient. The therapist should be knowledgeable about the anorectic illness and the therapeutic principles; open and nonevasive; intuitive, patient, and noncritical; and able to instill trust and confidence. In addition, the therapist should have a mode of relatedness that conveys empathy for and tolerance of painful emotions and challenges to treatment. Above all, the therapist must evidence a genuine spontaneity, humor, and flair for the dramatic. From a family therapy perspective, Sargant and colleagues (1985) have also identified the qualities of the therapist. In addition to those already mentioned by the other authors, they enumerated such skills as being comfortable with creating and escalating conflicts until resolution, able to direct or not to at appropriate times, able to focus on one issue even to the point of being unfair to one family member, and able to relate to both men and women in the family. These recommendations all make intuitive sense, and they all concur with one another: The therapist should be open, skillful, truthful, patient, tolerant, and able to relate well to an eating-disorder patient and her family.

However, research on the therapeutic qualities of a therapist has found them to be elusive. Beutler, Crago, and Arizmendi (1986) and Orlinsky and Howard (1986) have summarized recent research in therapist qualities, which may be roughly divided into "extra-therapy characteristics" and "therapy-specific characteristics." The former include such variables as age, gender, ethnicity, socioeconomic status, personality patterns, emotional well-being, and attitudes and values, while the latter include such variables as professional training and experience, therapeutic style and intervention skills, and relationship attitudes and attributes. Research on the therapeutic effects of extra-therapy characteristics has produced conflicting results; this is not surprising, since different patients probably relate well to different therapists. Of relevance to eating-disorder patients is the finding that adolescent female patients often prefer young female therapists, particularly those of a similar ethnic and socioeconomic background. Therapists such as Boskind-Lodahl (1976) and Palazzoli (1978) have always held that female therapists work better with eating-disorder patients, although psychoanalysts such as Rampling (1978) and Szyrynski (1973) have recommended male therapists. Practically all the research suggests that an emotionally healthy therapist is more likely to elicit a good outcome than an emotionally disturbed one. This issue may be relevant, since apparently more individuals who have had a personal history of an eating disorder are seeking to become therapists. It is unclear whether a recovered anorectic or bulimic is more or less effective as a therapist than someone without such a history. The therapist's personal attitude toward the current emphasis on slimness is obviously relevant to the treatment of the eating disorders, and it makes good clinical sense that someone who is overly weight conscious should probably not work with an eating-disorder patient. It is unclear what effect a non-weight-conscious but overweight therapist might have on the treatment process.

Regarding the therapy-specific characteristics, research has indicated that greater therapist experience may be related to positive outcome, but the findings regarding other characteristics, such as intervention style and theoretical orientation, are conflicting. In terms of the therapist's relational style, recent research certainly indicates that poor outcome may occur if the patient perceives the therapist to be hostile and critical. In contrast, patients generally do better if they perceive their therapist as engaged and empathic. Therapists who are perceived to be warm, accepting, and credible also tend to produce better outcomes. Although not overwhelming or consistent, there is some evidence to suggest that therapist–patient dissimilarity in terms of personality and relational style may affect outcome favorably. If so, this may support the contention of Strober and Yager (1985) that the therapist who is humorous, open, and spontaneous may be best suited for an adolescent anorectic who lacks such qualities.

I believe that because the above-mentioned studies were conducted only on competent therapists (whether formally trained or not), they have failed to identify the non-therapeutic qualities in a therapist. It is hard to imagine that incompetent therapists could have been included in such studies, or if they were, that they would not strive to behave more appropriately under scrutiny. While the earlier optimism in the power of therapist genuineness, empathy, and warmth has waned, their relevance for the treatment of eating-disorder patients should not be overlooked, particularly when a clinician is seeking to build a treatment team. It is common experience that some clinicians are much more likely than others to become locked in a battle of wills over management issues, such as how many cups of coffee a patient can have at each meal. I believe that one of the most important factors of success in the treatment of eating disorders is a dedicated and skillful team. Those seeking to build a treatment team will do well to wait for the right person to come along.

Engaging the Patient and Family as Collaborators

In the case of an adolescent patient, the initial contact with the clinic is usually made not by the patient but by a parent or someone concerned about her condition. A clinic staff member will then conduct a telephone intake interview at this point, discussing the main presenting problems with the person making the referral. An appointment is then made, at which point it is important for the clinician to explain clearly the purpose of the initial consultation. The clinician should also make sure that the patient herself is aware of this referral and of the purpose of the initial meeting. If the patient is living at home, the family should know about the referral unless the patient specifically forbids it. The clinic staff should request that all family members who live with the patient attend the initial consultation so that a complete evaluation can be made.

For a patient resistant to the idea of treatment, actually bringing her to the consultation may pose a problem. Some families may be tempted to trick her into attending, a ploy that is almost always disastrous in the long run. It is better to encourage a resistant patient to attend a support group, which may help her change her mind about treatment. The family should also be encouraged to attend a support group, since they may benefit from the experiences of other families in dealing with a resistant patient.

Patients usually arrive at the initial consultation with some apprehension, embarrassment, and resistance. Many clinicians have pointed out the importance of engaging the patient and family during the initial meeting, particularly during the first few minutes (Casper, 1982; Strober & Yager, 1985). Johnson and Connors (1987) seem to proceed with a structured interview, covering many areas of assessment, after the initial few minutes of the session. Strober and Yager (1985) defer assessment until later, after comprehensive discussion of the disorder with the patient and the family. I prefer the latter approach, sometimes deferring an extensive, semistructured interview until the second or third session if I detect resistance in the patient or family. I have already described my standard diagnostic approach in Chapter 5, and this diagnostic interview serves also to engage the patient and family in the majority of cases. However, sometimes the patient may express some reluctance to be seen together with the family, and I will then see her alone. I generally begin by acknowledging that, as far as I understand, there seems to be an eating problem. I then ask her how she feels about coming for the consultation. Most likely she will then be able to describe some of her eating difficulties, and I then proceed to discuss her actual experience of eating or her perception of weight. A compassionate and collaborative attitude and use of the patient's language are essential (Orbach, 1985). After the basic facts have been established, I affirm the importance of being thin and special and in control but at the same time indicate that her behavior may lead to serious complications. I explain the effects of starvation and outline the course of the illness. I also relate the illness to the tasks of adolescence and the conflicting role of women in society. I then describe the treatment program, assuring the patient that her specialness and control will not be taken away and that treatment will be a collaborative effort. I explain that I will therefore assiduously avoid forcing any treatment on her, such as tube feeding or hyperalimentation, unless definite indications arise.

To digress briefly, I have found it necessary to seek involuntary treatment in only a few instances for young, severely ill anorectic patients, an experience in common with that of Crisp (1980). In all such cases, the patients' inpatient stay after commitment was uneventful and weight gain was satisfactory. More important, most of them found the treatment to be a helpful experience and went on to maintain recovery. Of course, in younger patients (below the age of 16 for the state of Pennsylvania) commitment for involuntary treatment is not necessary, provided their parents give consent for treatment. The need to gain the patients' collaboration is, however, even greater in these cases.

Since most adolescent patients live with their families and the illness therefore always impinges on other family members, I ask for the patient's permission to meet with her family. It is essential to engage the family as a collaborator if treatment is not to be undermined. I almost never see the family without the patient. Even the most reluctant patient will agree to be seen with her family if the reasons for the family interview are carefully explained and if she is reassured of confidentiality; that is, what she has told me will not be reported to the parents. The joint meeting is spent in discussing the illness in general and answering the parents' concerns and questions. I usually try to deflect intrusive questions (e.g., "But why is she doing this to herself?") with such statements as, "Well, generally people starve themselves because they want to be thin and to be in control, and the pressure on women to be thin nowadays is so tremendous." If I feel that a patient is ready to enter into discussion with the parents, I may say, "Why don't you ask her." After explaining the effects of starvation, the course of the illness, the possible complications, and the treatment program, I usually recommend books to the patient and family, such as *The Golden Cage* (Bruch, 1978) or *Anorexia Nervosa:*

Let Me Be (Crisp, 1980), and give them handouts that briefly describe the illness and its treatment. I also recommend a support group if the patient does not already attend one. A physical examination is scheduled, and blood and urine tests are ordered.

This process of engagement may take a few sessions or even longer. As explained in Chapter 5, I sometimes assign the same therapist for both the individual patient and the family. Regarding resistant patients who cannot go beyond the first session, I always inform them that they can contact me whenever they feel ready for treatment; quite a few have done so, sometimes after a gap of months or even years.

Breaking Confidentiality

The very ill patient who both refuses treatment and refuses to give permission to contact the family presents the dilemma of whether to break patient confidentiality. In the few instances in which I have done so, usually in the case of a college student living away from home, I have abided by the following rules: (1) consult with a colleague to confirm that the patient's clinical condition is sufficiently serious to warrant immediate treatment; (2) inform the patient of the intent to contact her family and the reasons for doing so; (3) contact the family by telephone in the presence of the patient; and (4) document clearly in the case record the patient's clinical condition, the consultation with a colleague, the discussion with the patient, the reasons for contacting the family despite her refusal to give permission, and the result of the discussion with the family. In the few cases in which I have done this, the family then came for a joint session with the patient.

TREATING ANOREXIA NERVOSA

A baffling array of treatments have been advocated for anorexia nervosa in the last 30 years. In 1960, Dally and Sargant described the use of chlorpromazine and modified insulin as a new treatment for the illness, and in the subsequent years behavioral therapy (Blinder, Freeman, & Stunkard, 1970), family therapy (Minuchin, 1974), and hyperalimentation (Maloney & Farrell, 1980) have in turn been accorded the same honor. The list of treatment of choice is equally lengthy, ranging from tube feeding (Williams, 1958) to psychoanalysis (Wilson, 1983). Unfortunately, the writings sometimes either reflect the exasperation of a therapist trapped in a battle of wills with the patient (Bruch, 1973) or demonstrate an ignorance of the long-term outcome of the disorder or a confusion regarding treatment goals (Russell, 1977b). Thus, for instance, rapid weight gain can certainly occur with behavioral modification, tube feeding, or hyperalimentation, but it does not affect long-term outcome and it induces fear and a feeling of loss of control in the patient. Insistent, even strident, claims for the proven efficacy of family therapy (e.g., Minuchin et al., 1978; Sargent et al., 1985) or psychoanalysis (Hogan, 1983; Wilson, 1983) belie the fact that the data presented have major methodological flaws.

As already mentioned, recent research has clarified a number of treatment issues for anorexia nervosa, although there has been no major breakthrough. The following discussion is organized according to the major issues that confront a clinician who encounters a patient with anorexia nervosa.

The Treatment Setting

After the initial consultation, the clinician has to decide whether to treat the patient as an inpatient or as an outpatient. While opinions differ, most clinicians would probably recommend inpatient treatment if one or more of the following exists: a low body weight, physical complications, severe depression or suicidal feeling or behavior, and failure of outpatient treatment. Clinical experience suggests that a patient who is not vomiting or purging and has maintained a stable, albeit low, body weight for many months may be treated successfully as an outpatient provided further weight loss or complications do not occur.

If body weight has fallen below 70% of the average (Casper, 1982; Garfinkel & Garner, 1982; Morgan, Purgold, & Welbourne, 1983) or if weight loss has been rapid, then inpatient treatment is usually recommended. Acute cardiac failure due to loss of left ventricular mass is a serious complication, the possibility of which a clinician cannot afford to ignore. Nutritional treatment for a very emaciated patient is best carried out in a hospital because of the risks of serious complications that may occur on refeeding, such as acute gastric dilatation or generalized peripheral edema. In addition to being life-saving, inpatient treatment may foster an otherwise fragile treatment alliance and allow the initiation of meaningful psychotherapy (Bruch, 1982; Casper, 1987; Minuchin et al., 1978). Sometimes a bulimic anorectic at a higher weight may require inpatient treatment, since the electrolyte disturbances resulting from vomiting and purging may lead to acute cardiac failure. Other complications, such as acute gastric dilatation, esophageal bleeding, or massive peripheral edema, are emergencies that require immediate inpatient treatment. Dysphoria is common in anorectics, and some fulfill criteria for major depression. Most patients are not severely depressed, but a psychotic episode is probably best managed on an inpatient basis. Suicide is a distinct possibility, and a patient who has suicidal ideations or has made previous attempts should be managed as an inpatient. Finally, weight loss during outpatient treatment often signals the need for inpatient treatment.

As already mentioned, not all clinicians agree with the above indications for inpatient treatment. Reinhart, Kenna, and Succop (1972) recommend hospitalization only to effect a brief separation of the child from "an anxious and frightened environment." These authors also recommend hospitalization if the patient is frightened because she feels her dieting is out of control or if she becomes psychotic. They claim good results in almost all their 32 pediatric patients, but it is unclear how many were treated also as inpatients. As will be discussed later, such claims are notoriously difficult to evaluate.

In my view, weight restoration is best carried out on a unit that has an experienced staff and usually has more than one or two eating-disorder patients at any one time. The team should be able to conduct behavioral therapy, nursing care, and psychotherapy competently. The team should also be able to anticipate manipulation and deception and quickly defuse such situations with tact and patience. However, for practical reasons admission to such a unit is not always feasible, and many patients are admitted to general psychiatric adolescent wards. Anorectics may find the interaction with non-eating-disorder adolescents with different social backgrounds and difficulties interesting and perhaps even beneficial (Strober & Yager, 1985). However, determining the right mix of patients on an adolescent unit is always difficult, and because of their nonassertive nature anorectics may sometimes be victimized by those with a conduct disorder. It is certainly my experience that parents and patients usually prefer treatment on an eating-disorder unit, where the patient does not feel isolated and different.

Sometimes patients are admitted to a general pediatric or medical ward for the treatment of acute physical complications or severe emaciation. Reinhart and colleagues (1972) recommend that in these circumstances the psychiatrist take responsibility for both the physical and psychological management, since "there can only be one master" (p. 118). While this may be the ideal situation, most therapists probably end up working in collaboration with a pediatrician or an internist. Minuchin and colleagues (1978) have written extensively about the role of the physician as a member of the treatment team for anorexia nervosa, providing the following scenario: After full evaluation, the physician and the therapist jointly meet with the patient and the family; the physician then proceeds to review the physical findings and inform the patient and family of the seriousness of the situation; further, the physician states quite forcefully that there is no physical cause for the symptoms and that the family should now work with the therapist to help the patient return to normal physical health; the physician also determines the target weight and suggests appropriate daily calorie intake and rate of weight gain. Thus the physician is cast in a role of authority and power in the treatment of anorectic patients, and Minuchin and colleagues suggest that close collaboration with the physician is essential. On a medical ward, many patients are probably given tube feeding or hyperalimentation in order to facilitate weight gain. While I am in general against the use of such coercive techniques for reasons to be described later, I do not have hard evidence to suggest that they are contraindicated and thus acknowledge that good results may sometimes occur (e.g., Williams, 1958).

The major difficulty of admission to a general medical or surgical ward is, in my opinion, the lack of experience of the ward staff in the management of these patients. Tinker and Ramer (1983) documented several incidents of staff subversion of the treatment of several anorectic patients admitted to an adolescent medical ward, including the following: the staff's making critical comments about patients' food choice and issuing unauthorized increase of their caloric intake;

purposeful avoidance of interaction with the patients; and, in one incident, asking an anorectic to watch another patient having an epileptic seizure in order to teach her what a real illness was. It is, of course, possible that with better training and supervision such countertherapeutic interactions could be prevented, but it is unclear how many hospitals are prepared to implement such training and supervision.

While most therapists agree that inpatient treatment is indicated for the very ill anorectic, opinions differ on the goals of inpatient treatment. At one extreme, Crisp (1967, 1980) has recommended that inpatient treatment be instituted until the patient reaches "target weight" (see below for details) and then continue for at least another 2 weeks, during which there is a gradual increase in the patient's autonomy and activity. At the other extreme, Mintz (1983) has recommended that inpatient treatment be as short as possible, the goal being to restore the patient to a "modicum of health" so that outpatient psychoanalysis can continue. While Crisp has published extensive data on his work, Mintz and other psychoanalysts who share similar views (e.g., Wilson 1983) have not.

Treatment Goals

Most clinicians would agree that the first treatment goal is weight restoration, since the self-imposed starvation is responsible for many of the symptoms of the disorder. Not only is weight restoration lifesaving, it may also improve the patient's morbid mental attitudes. The latter may seem paradoxical, but many clinicians have documented an improvement in the fat phobia in conjunction with weight gain (Garfinkel & Garner, 1982; Morgan & Russell, 1975). The second goal is the establishment of healthy eating habits in the context of restoring the patient's nutritional status (Huse & Lucas, 1985). A third treatment goal, which many consider to be primary, is to change the patient's pursuit of thinness and her deficits in the regulation of her mood and her behaviors. A fourth goal is the treatment of physical complications and concomitant psychiatric symptoms, if present. A fifth goal is the prevention of relapse, since apparently 50% of patients will experience a relapse within 1 year of discharge from the hospital. Finally, bulimic anorectics require specific treatments for their binge-and-purge behavior.

The clinician must recognize, however, that these treatment goals may not be applicable to a chronic patient who has had many hospitalizations. Aggressive treatment for a chronic patient may precipitate depression and suicide (Crisp, 1980), and great clinical acumen is needed for her management, which will be briefly discussed later (see section "Treating Chronic Patients"). Moreover, not all clinicians accept the importance of nutritional restoration as a specific treatment goal. Orbach (1985), for instance, recommends making an agreement with the patient early on in treatment that if she agrees not to go below her weight at the initiation of treatment then the therapist will not intervene with her actual intake. Reinhart and colleagues (1972) repeatedly tell the patient and parents that as clinicians their primary concern is her angry and hopeless feelings, which cause her not to eat and which they will deal with by psychotherapy, and that they will only focus on her eating behavior if they believe it is necessary. Psychoanalysts such as Wilson (1983) avoid all discussions of the need for weight gain.

In the absence of properly conducted treatment studies it is impossible to be dogmatic about treatment goals. However, practically all clinicians who have treated large numbers of patients have made similar recommendations to those just outlined (Andersen, 1985; Bruch, 1973; Crisp, 1980; Garfinkel & Garner, 1982; Goodsitt, 1985; Russell, 1970; Strober & Yager, 1985). Further, clinicians who deemphasize weight gain in treatment have rarely published their findings in sufficient detail to allow for objective evaluation. Finally, since the starvation and emaciation are directly responsible for many of the symptoms, common sense suggests that it should be dealt with directly in the majority of patients.

Weight Restoration

Efforts to restore body weight may be grouped into five main categories: (1) nursing care combined with nutritional treatment and some restriction of activities; (2) behavior modification; (3) coercive treatment, such as tube feeding and hyperalimentation; (4) psychotherapy; and (5) pharmacotherapy. Needless to say, clinicians often use these approaches in various combinations.

It may be surprising to the uninitiated that weight restoration is in fact one of the least problematic treatment tasks for anorexia nervosa. Weight restoration is usually successful in at least 85% of patients, provided the following principles are fulfilled:

1. Weight restoration occurs in conjunction with other treatments, such as individual and family therapy, so that the patient does not feel that eating and weight gain are the only goals of treatment.
2. The patient trusts the treatment team and believes that she will not be allowed to become overweight.
3. The patient's fear of loss of control is contained; this may be accomplished by having her eat frequent, smaller meals (e.g., four to six times per day, with 400 to 500 calories per meal) so as to produce a gradual but steady weight gain (e.g., an average of 0.2 kg/day).
4. A member of the nursing staff is present during mealtimes to encourage the patient to eat and to discuss her fears and anxiety about eating and weight gain.
5. Gradual weight gain rather than the amount of food eaten is regularly monitored, and the result is made known to the patient; thus the patient should be weighed at regular intervals, and she should know whether she has gained or lost weight.
6. Some negative and positive reinforcements exist, such as the use of a graduated level of activity and bedrest, whether or not these reinforcements are formally conceptualized as behavior modification techniques, so that the patient may thereby learn that she can control not only her behavior but also the consequence of her behavior.
7. The patient's self-defeating behavior, such as surreptitious vomiting or purging, is confronted and controlled.
8. The dysfunctional conflict between the patient and the family about eating and food is not reenacted in the hospital; or if the pattern is to be reenacted in a therapeutic lunch session, the purpose is clearly defined.

Clinicians treating large numbers of anorectic patients have reported encouraging results for the vast majority of patients when these principles of weight restoration are used. Such findings should allow at least the following conclusions to be drawn: (1) that a carefully planned, structured inpatient treatment program implemented consistently by a competent treatment team is effective for restoring weight in the vast majority of cases; (2) that coercive treatments (such as tube feeding or hyperalimentation), overrestrictive measures (such as locking rooms and depriving patients of basic necessities), and pharmacotherapy are usually unnecessary; and (3) that such measures should be used, if at all, only in refractory cases or when definite clinical indications are present.

Obviously these principles encompass different interventions, and unless a "dismantling" technique is used, it is at present impossible to say whether any or all of these interventions are necessary or equally effective. Each technique is discussed below.

Nursing Care and Dietary Treatment

Nursing care and dietary treatment are the bedrock of many inpatient programs, although their therapeutic efficacy is not always acknowledged. Until recently dietary treatment was instituted with the primary purpose of bringing the patient's body weight up to a normal level, while nursing care was the main component of the milieu in which the dietary treatment was instituted.

Several authors have described their nutritional treatment approach (Crisp, 1967; Garfinkel & Garner, 1982; Powers & Powers, 1984; Russell, 1970). In principle a patient should be given a balanced diet so that she can gain on average about 1 to 2 kilograms (2 to 4 pounds) per week. More rapid weight gain may be gratifying to the clinician but may induce fear and a feeling of loss of control in the patient. Although both Crisp and Russell apparently placed their patients on a high-calorie diet right from the beginning, it is probably advisable to start with a moderate amount of calories (1,000 to 1,500 calories) so that the complications of rapid refeeding in an emaciated patient, such as acute gastric dilatation or massive peripheral edema, may be avoided. The caloric value of the diet can be gradually increased after the first few days. More frequent but smaller meals (for instance, six meals per day of 400–600 calories each) may help avoid the sense of distention after eating and be less frightening to the patient. A large meal may induce greater consumption (Agras, Barlow, Chapin, Abel, & Leitenberg, 1974) but, again, may induce fear and a sense of loss of control. It is also not conducive to the development of normal eating habits: A patient probably finds it more reassuring if she finishes all of her meals and gains an average of 1 to 2 kilograms per week than if she has to leave half of her meals unfinished in order to gain the same amount. Some clinicians advocate the use of liquid food supplements (Powers & Powers, 1984; Russell, 1970), but the indications for their use are obscure, and, again, they probably do not encourage the development of normal eating habits. A dietician who meets regularly with the patient is always helpful, not only in helping the patient make proper food choices but also in providing her with nutritional education, a point to which we will return later.

A team of experienced, skillful, and patient nurses is usually given the task of encouraging the patient to complete her meals and of providing supervision so that she does not discard her food surreptitiously or engage in other weight-reducing measures. The nursing staff should therefore remain close at hand as the patient eats, to persuade and cajole her to finish her food and to distract her from any anxieties regarding eating and weight gain. The patient will often complain of feeling full or nauseous after eating, and a nurse may reassure her that the feelings may be related to the slow gastric emptying that occurs in anorexia nervosa and that such feelings should disappear in time. A nurse who suspects that the patient is secretly purging or discarding food should confront her gently by saying, in the words of Russell (1977b), "I know that you are really an honest and truthful person but I also know that your illness may compel you to do things which are not in your nature, especially when you become anxious about putting on weight" (p. 282). Following this explanation the nurse may carry out a room search, but this should always be conducted in the presence of the patient. Educational and supportive psychotherapy should be given by the nurse when necessary. The patient may need repeated reassurance that she will not be allowed to become fat. As the patient gains weight, her anxiety will be focused on the fat accumulation in her abdomen, her buttocks, or her thighs, and the nurse should explain to her that there is indeed a tendency for the weight to go first to these body parts but that in time it will redistribute itself. It is of interest to note that Berkman (Griffin, Frazier, Robinson, & Johnson, 1957), a Mayo Clinic physician who began treating anorectics in the 1930s, essentially used the same educational and supportive approach. In order to prevent staff splitting and facilitate communication, it is probably wise to limit the size of the nursing team, and, if possible, to include only full-time nurses on the team. Crisp (Crisp et al., 1985) assigns an "individual assessor" (i.e., the equivalent of a primary nurse) to each patient, who is encouraged to discuss all nutritional and weight issues with this person.

At the beginning of treatment, activities are usually restricted to varying degrees. Crisp confines the patient to bedrest in a cubicle on the ward until she reaches target weight. He argues that it symbolizes the restrictions and confinements of the illness, although others may see its significance in behavior modification terms. Russell (1977b) simply confines the patient to the ward without specific mention of bedrest. A consistent and coherent policy on activity level should be developed for each individual treatment program.

As already mentioned, the main concern of most authors is to encourage the patient to eat so as to gain weight to a normal level. However, it is by no means certain that normal eating habits will develop spontaneously in conjunction with weight gain (Huse & Lucas, 1985; Wilson, Touyz, O'Connor, & Beumont, 1985). In fact, practically all the follow-up studies indicate that abnormal eating patterns may persist even in those who have regained normal weight. However, very little has been written specifically on the treatment of abnormal eating habits. Huse and Lucas (1985) described in some detail an educational approach that deserves more study. They define the goals of dietary treatment as: (1) helping the patient understand her nutritional needs for growth and tissue maintenance and how these needs can be met by food, and (2) helping the patient understand her energy needs to reach and maintain an appropriate body weight. To achieve these goals, the dietician first takes a careful dietary history in order to understand the patient's eating pattern, identify her areas of strength and deficiency, and build rapport and understanding. Nutritional education is given in the context of designing a diet with sufficient calories. When a more healthy eating pattern is established, discussions then center on increasing the caloric content and identifying weight-increase expectations. Finally, when goal weight is attained, a maintenance diet plan is implemented. Others (e.g., Garner, Rockert, Olmsted, Johnson, & Coscina, 1985) also include educating the patient regarding the dangers of laxative or diuretic abuse, purchasing nutritional foods, and the importance of eating a variety of foods. Hall and Crisp (1987) have recently compared the efficacy of 12 sessions of dietary advice with 12 sessions of combined individual and family therapy. Sessions were held at weekly to biweekly intervals. Outcome was largely similar at the end of treatment and at 1-year follow-up: Both treatments were associated with significant weight gain as well as improvement in general adjustment. Social and sexual adjustments, however, were somewhat superior for the psychotherapy group. Unfortunately, there was some overlap in the content of the two treatments, and thus improvement in the nutritional group could not be ascribed definitively to dietary counseling. Obviously, dietary treatment needs further study.

There is no agreement of what constitutes a target weight for anorectics, although most clinicians probably use a low average weight for height, age, and sex as a general guide. Crisp (1980; Crisp et al., 1985) has repeatedly argued that the target weight should be the appropriate weight at age of onset of the illness, on the grounds that the patient has to be reexposed to the issues, symbolized by body weight, that precipitated the illness. Collins, Hodas, and Liebman (1983), while using age-appropriate weight as the target, nevertheless discharge their patients after they have gained 50% of the weight gain needed to achieve target weight. It is unclear which approach is more effective in the long run but I have been using Crisp's approach.

Some clinicians determine the target weight without prior consultation with the patient (e.g., Crisp et al., 1985; Russell, 1977b), while others negotiate with the patient (e.g., Minuchin, Rosman, & Baker, 1978). It is unclear which is more effective, but it is important to remember that patients will always bargain for a lower weight; thus firmness is always necessary. Some set a specific target weight (e.g., Crisp et al., 1985), while others use a range (e.g., Garfinkel & Garner, 1982). Again, it is unclear which is more effective. Clinicians should therefore be guided by their own preferences on these issues.

Behavior Modification

In the 1960s single-case studies began to demonstrate the effectiveness of behavior therapy as a means of helping anorectic patients gain weight. Studies with a more substantial number of patients began to appear in the 1970s (Agras et al., 1974; Bhanji & Thompson, 1974; Blinder et al., 1970; Halmi, Powers, & Cunningham 1975). Because of its proven efficacy at inducing short-term weight gain, most clinicians now probably incorporate some form of behavioral modification into the treatment of an emaciated anorectic patient. Elkin, Hersen, Eisler, and Williams (1973) and Agras, Barlow, Chapin, Abel, and Leitenberg (1974) found that information feedback, reinforcement, and size of meal all increase caloric consumption and rate of weight gain. Information feedback is usually achieved by having the patient keep a weight chart, since techniques directed at weight gain are probably more effective than those that focus on eating habits per se (Touyz, Beumont, & Glaun, 1984). The patients are usually weighed once a day or once or twice a week, and the frequency of weighing apparently has no effect on the overall amount of weight gain. Since body weight fluctuates during the day, weighing is probably best carried out in the morning, after the patient has used the bathroom and before breakfast. Incidentally, physicians such as Crisp and Russell, who do not conceptualize treatment in behavioral modification terms, have been using regular weighing for a long time.

Positive reinforcements contingent on weight gain are always used and include increased physical and social activity and visiting privileges. Negative reinforcements, such as bedrest and isolation in the bedroom, may also be used. Tube feeding and hyperalimentation can obviously be regarded as negative reinforcers; as already mentioned, they are rarely necessary. An individualized approach with a detailed behavioral analysis is perhaps important, since patients differ in their preferences and response. However, this may create practical difficulties for a team that is treating more than a few patients at any one time. Furthermore, Touyz and colleagues (1984) found no difference in mean weekly weight gain between patients in strict and lenient operant-conditioning programs. The strict program consisted of bedrest and an individualized schedule of reinforcers for each 0.5 kg of weight gain. The lenient program consisted of a contract stipulating that a minimum gain of 1.5 kg/week would allow the patient to move freely around the unit; otherwise, she would spend the following week in bed. Although assignment to the two treatments was not randomized, the findings argue for the routine use of a lenient structure rather than a restrictive one.

A large meal may induce greater consumption and therefore usually also greater weight gain (Agras et al., 1974; Elkin et al., 1973), but as already discussed in the previous section on Nursing Care and

Dietary Treatment, it may not encourage the development of normal eating habits, and it may induce fear and a feeling of loss of control in the patient. Furthermore, rapid refeeding in an emaciated patient may lead to serious complications, and large meals should be avoided, at least during the initial stages of treatment.

In a study designed to compare behavior modification and milieu therapy, Eckert, Goldberg, Halmi, Casper, and Davis (1979) randomly assigned 81 anorexia nervosa patients to behavior modification or milieu therapy for 35 days. There was no overall significant difference in weight gain between the two groups. Since both groups gained an average of 1.0 kg/week, it would appear that behavior modification conferred no additional benefit over a milieu program in the treatment of acute anorexia nervosa. Furthermore, the long-term outcome of the two groups of patients was apparently not different.

Many anorectic patients complain of social anxiety and diffidence, therefore social-skills training may be useful. Pillay and Crisp (1981) found that 12 sessions of social-skills training indeed reduced anxiety and depression, but such short-term improvement was not sustained at follow-up, nor did it prevent weight loss after discharge. Perhaps a more intensive program is necessary to produce change; clearly, more research is needed.

Finally, systematic desensitization has been used in a small number of patients to induce weight gain and to desensitize them to the fear of fatness and fear of comments from peers regarding their weight (Hallsten, 1965; Ollendick, 1979; Schnurer, Rubin, & Roy, 1973). Results seemed promising in terms of short-term weight gain. The technique may be useful as a treatment for fear of fatness in patients who have regained normal weight, but unfortunately there has been no recent research on the use of systematic desensitization for anorexia nervosa.

In summary, behavior modification is effective in inducing short-term weight gain. Unfortunately, most of the earlier studies conceptualized this as the only valid treatment goal, and they primarily focused on how much weight was gained by a patient per week. Recent research has demonstrated not only that the rate of weight gain is inconsequential in terms of long-term outcome but also that successful weight restoration during hospitalization is a relatively weak predictor of long-term prognosis (Hsu, 1988). Furthermore, many studies were conducted with the use of inappropriate reinforcers, such as intense and unrestricted physical activity or meetings with the dietician, or with outdated concepts, such as the belief that a low-frequency activity (eating) will increase if rewarded by permission to indulge in a high-frequency behavior (overactivity). Such ill-conceived ideas may have persisted to this day, and clinicians using behavior therapy will do well to think through the basic principles.

Individual Psychotherapy

Since the basic psychopathology in anorexia nervosa is a morbid fear of fatness, psychotherapy aimed at resolving this fear and other related psychological disturbances should at least theoretically provide the patient with the best chance of lasting recovery (Russell, 1970). Practically all the researchers have emphasized the importance of psychotherapy, but few have attempted to prove its efficacy. The absence of hard data does not mean that psychotherapy is ineffective; rather it means that for now the therapist should be open and flexible and be guided by experience and common sense. It is, however, comforting to note that recent writings on the psychotherapy of anorexia nervosa are in broad agreement on several themes, despite the fact that they reflect widely different theoretical perspectives.

Earlier psychoanalytic interpretation of anorexia nervosa considered it to be related to a rejection of female genital sexuality and oral impregnation fantasies by means of starvation. This was thought to be accompanied by a regression to pregenital defense mechanisms in the face of conflict centered on primitive sadistic and cannibalistic oral fantasies. Sours (1980) suggests that the onset of anorexia nervosa during early adolescence is related to fixation at the phallic-oedipal or late separation–individuation phase, with the anorectic symptoms being mobilized as a defense against emerging sexual drives. Onset in late adolescence, in Sours's view, is related to fixation at the symbiotic and early separation–individuation phase, with the symptoms related more to ego defects. Object-relations theories consider it to be related to the introjection and repression of a bad object consequent upon the early ambivalent relationship with an aggressively overprotective, unresponsive, castrating, domineering, or controlling mother. On a more superficial level, it is generally recognized that starvation serves as an expression of hostility, control, and aggression toward the family. As already mentioned in Chapter 4, these ideas lack empirical support.

The primary task of the analyst is to make interpretations with reference to both the actual transference that occurs in therapy and the earlier experiences that have been repressed. Bruch (1973; 1982), Casper (1987), Crisp (1980), Garner and Bemis (1982), Halmi (1983), Minuchin (1974), and Palazzoli (1974) have all found the traditional psychoanalytic approach rather ineffective.

Because the anorectic is usually an adolescent in the process of striving for individuation and identity formation, many authors have conceptualized the illness in terms of developmental aberrations. Bruch has written extensively on the theory and practice of psychotherapy in anorexia nervosa (Bruch, 1962, 1973, 1982, 1985), and her writings have perhaps been the most influential of those by psychotherapists. She emphasizes an evocative, fact-finding approach by paying careful attention to the patient's feelings, sensations, and ideas. This is in contrast to the traditional interpretive approach, which may reinforce the patient's feeling that someone else knows what she herself does not know. Bruch recommends initiating treatment by giving a dynamic explanation of the meaning of the illness: that the preoccupation with eating and weight serves as a cover-up for the underlying problems and severe self-doubts. The patient is then invited to express her feelings and wants, and her right, even duty, to do so is spelled out. Her need to behave and be perfect, her self-doubt and self-belittling, her belief that her worth depends on others' approval, and her basic distrust despite the apparent need to please are systematically dealt with. Since Bruch conceptualizes anorexia nervosa as a misguided quest for identity, the development of a new personality is the ultimate goal of her treatment.

Crisp (1980; Crisp et al., 1985) has long maintained that anorexia nervosa is a psychobiological regression that occurs in the face of mounting adolescent conflict that the illness serves to avert, both for the individual and for her family. Crisp's therapeutic approach is eclectic: While in general he uses a psychodynamic, interpretive approach, he also uses nutritional counseling, social-skills training, and sexual therapy. Crisp's writings are, however, more concerned with the main themes of the disorder than with the actual therapeutic techniques. Strober and Yager (1985) have also emphasized the treatment of anorexia nervosa from a developmental perspective.

Garfinkel and Garner (1982) and Garner and Bemis (1982) have used a cognitive approach that involves teaching the patient to examine the validity of her beliefs on a moment-to-moment basis. The patient's cognitive processes, such as selective abstraction, over-generalization, magnification, dichotomous thinking, personalization, and superstitious thinking, are first examined and defined, and each is then systematically challenged so that her automatic thoughts and assumptions may be modified. These authors have also used a more psychoeducational approach (Garner, Rockert, Olmsted, Johnson, & Coscina, 1985), in which such themes as the cultural context of the emphasis on slimness, the effects of starvation on behavior, weight regulation and set-point theory, the metabolic adaptations to prolonged dieting, the ineffectiveness of purging, and the metabolic consequences of refeeding are extensively discussed with the patient. This model of focusing on the proximal causal and maintaining variables relies heavily on the cognitive therapy model developed by Beck (1976), in which the therapist actively encourages the patient to identify her cognitions and beliefs, invites her to examine them rationally, and challenges her on their validity.

Goodsitt (1985) has described an approach based on the view that anorectics have a deficit in the self. By "self," Goodsitt means the capacity of the psyche to maintain self-esteem and cohesiveness and to regulate tensions and moods. Goodsitt believes that the anorectic's sense of ineffectiveness and impaired awareness of feelings and sensations are best explained by defects in the ego or self. He therefore goes beyond confrontative and interpretive interventions, actively filling in the patient's ego deficits by allowing himself to be used as a "transitional" or "self" object by the patient. He therefore actively soothes and calms the patient; he explains, exhorts, teaches, prescribes, and evokes. He is a parent, guide, teacher, and coach. He is, in fact, "managing" rather than "interpreting" the transference, and, through using him as a transitional object, the patient learns to regulate her inner tensions. Furthermore, through encouraging the patient to get in touch with her inner experiences, the therapist helps her integrate her external behavior with her inner experiences and feelings. Clearly, therapists may do many of these things without subscribing to Goodsitt's view on self-psychology, and Berkman (see Griffin et al., 1957), Levenkron (1983), and Reinhart (Reinhart et al., 1972), among others, have described much the same approach from entirely different theoretical perspectives.

Orbach (1985) takes a feminist view that anorexia nervosa is related to the psychological construction of femininity and the vicissitudes of passage from girlhood to womanhood in contemporary Western society. Aside from this perspective, Orbach's therapeutic approach is actually not very different from those thus far described. For instance, she emphasizes that the therapist should strive to make contact with the "pre-related" self of the patient. The importance of this point has been emphasized by all the aforementioned therapists, albeit in different terms.

Finally, many authors have discussed the difficult therapeutic task of altering the patient's fear of fatness. Garner, Rockert, Olmsted, Johnson, and Coscina (1985) suggest to the patient that she should live with it, recognizing that it is a part of the anorectic illness. Whenever this fear surfaces, she should simply blame it on the illness. Other therapists have suggested to the patient that the fear of fatness serves to cover up certain feelings or thoughts that she is unwilling to confront, and thus she is encouraged to focus her attention on such thoughts and feelings rather than on the weight phobia. Alternatively, systematic desensitization may be used to treat the weight phobia. However, the few published single-case reports (see Ollendick, 1979) have focused on intake and rate of weight gain rather than on fat phobia. The efficacy of this technique is therefore unknown, and in future studies a specific hierarchy for weight phobia should be constructed for desensitization. Wooley and Wooley (1985) have found experiential techniques to be useful in the treatment of disturbances of body image. Using imagery, art, and movement, they attempt to enhance the patient's awareness of her distortion of body image and its development. Experiential techniques are then used to help her gain a sense of control over her perceptions and feelings about her body, the final goal being the creation of a more positive body image.

In summary, recent writings on individual psychotherapy have focused on the patient's inward emptiness, denial and fear of personal needs, sense of ineffectiveness, low self-esteem, and self-hatred. The writings have also focused on the importance of helping the patient work through the normal adolescent developmental tasks. They emphasize the need of the therapist to educate, to modulate, to support, to evoke, to discuss, to challenge, to negotiate, to encourage, and to role-model.

Family Therapy

While many therapists have used some family therapy to treat anorectic patients (e.g., Bruch, 1982; Crisp, 1980; Garfinkel & Garner,
1982), Minuchin (1974; Minuchin et al., 1978) and Palazzoli (1978;
Palazzoli, Boscolo, Cecchin, & Prata, 1977) are perhaps the most
vociferous in their advocacy of family therapy as a primary treatment
for anorexia nervosa. Their writings make fascinating reading and
have offered promise of a radical, alternative form of treatment.
However, experience has indicated that family therapy is not the
panacea it was once thought to be. Nevertheless, it is a useful therapeutic tool, and its efficacy and indication need to be carefully
studied.

Minuchin and his colleagues take a systems perspective and
aim at changing the dysfunctional family structure, which, they postulate, reinforces the anorectic behavior in the patient. Family structure can be conceptualized in terms of hierarchy, subsystems, and
boundaries, and it governs the transactions between family members.
In the case of the anorectic family, such transactions are characterized
by enmeshment, overprotectiveness, rigidity, lack of conflict resolution, and involvement of the sick child in unresolved parental conflicts. Thus, in contrast to other investigators, Minuchin and his
colleagues emphasize the interpersonal rather than the intrapsychic
processes of anorexia nervosa. Their open-systems model, deemed
applicable to all psychosomatic illnesses, includes many parts, which
can be activated at any point and are dependent on each other.
Minuchin and his colleagues have, however, focused almost exclu-
sively in their writings on the treatment of the family, stating that
"when significant family interaction patterns are changed, significant
changes in the symptoms of the psychosomatic illness also occur"
(Minuchin et al., 1978, p. 21). From a developmental perspective, they
suggest that the anorectic family structure, with its inability to promote individual development or allow for open negotiation of affec-
tion, intimacy, and mutual respect, hinders the adolescent in her
growth and development. The goal of family therapy is therefore first
to unbalance the homeostatic dysfunctional transactional pattern and
then to reorganize the family structure around more open and
healthy communication. Minuchin and colleagues have described
techniques to join in collaboration with the family, enact dysfunc-

tional transactions, focus selectively on strategic issues, increase the intensity of conflict, define boundaries, delineate subsystems, establish complementarity of responsibility, and prescribe change. Sometimes they advocate the use of a family lunch session to bring into the open dysfunctional transactional patterns, "to transform the issue of an anorectic patient to the drama of a dysfunctional family" (Minuchin et al., 1978, p. 120). These issues are then confronted and dealt with. Throughout treatment the therapist focuses on the interactional process as well as the content of communication, and in practice many educational, strategic, behavioral, and paradoxical techniques are also used. More recently, Minuchin's colleagues have also used individual therapy in addition to family therapy (e.g., Sargent et al., 1985), particularly toward the final phase of treatment. The same therapist conducts both the individual and the family therapy, and the individual therapy is conducted primarily from a family perspective, although discussions of peer, school, and love relationships also occur. In individual sessions four approaches are used to help the patient with her family and individuation–separation issues: (1) developing methods to change how the family treats her; (2) minimizing her role in repetitive nonproductive interactions with the family; (3) recognizing and accepting the unchangeable aspects of the family; and (4) improving her social life outside of the family.

Palazzoli and her colleagues have used strategic and paradoxical interventions calculated to change the family dynamics without resorting to explanation, criticism, or any other verbal intervention. They believe that sometimes verbal requests for change can only stimulate the fear of change and strengthen the existing family interaction pattern. Their interventions are therefore not intended to promote insight, emotional release, or personal growth; instead, they are plans of action designed to replace old dysfunctional transactions. For instance, in one case described by Palazzoli and colleagues (1977) the therapists, after consulting with the entire treatment team (who had been observing the sessions behind a one-way mirror), prescribed the following ritual to a tightly knit family living under the "myth" that loyalty to members of the extended family clan should be maintained at any price: The nuclear family was to sit around the dining room table for 1 hour every other evening after dinner, with the front door locked and bolted; each member was to speak his or her mind about members of the extended family for 15 minutes or else was to remain silent; when a person was speaking, the other family members were to listen and remain silent. The purpose of the ritual was primarily to strengthen the nuclear family, allowing each individual member to voice criticisms of the clan without being labeled as disloyal or bad. More recently, perhaps in response to criticisms about the ambiguity of their approach, the Milan group (Palazzoli, Boscolo, Cecchin, and Prata, 1980; Cecchin, 1987) described three guidelines for the family therapist who is conducting the evaluation of the family: hypothesizing, circularity, and neutrality. Briefly stated, the therapist should generate a family-oriented working hypothesis from the referral material; test it out by eliciting data from each family member (typically by inviting one member to tell the clinician how he or she sees the relationship between two other members of the family); and maintain different alliances with each family member at different times of the session. Both Minuchin and Palazzoli have relied heavily on the help of a therapeutic team that observes the sessions behind a one-way mirror. At appropriate times during the session, the therapist conducting the family session consults with the team to get a sense of which direction to move toward.

Despite repeated claims that outcome studies have demonstrated the efficacy of family therapy (e.g., Minuchin et al., 1978; Rosman, Minuchin, Baker, & Liebman, 1977), it must be realized that the technique has not been adequately investigated by controlled studies. To the best of my knowledge, only one study exists that compares the efficacy of family therapy with individual therapy. Russell, Szmukler, Dare, and Eisler (1987) randomly assigned 57 anorectic and 23 bulimic anorectic patients to either family therapy or individual supportive therapy after they had had a period of inpatient treatment to restore their body weights to low-average levels. All the anorectics belonged to the restrictor (i.e., abstaining) subgroup, and they were further subdivided into three subgroups: (1) patients with a young age of onset (on or before the age of 18) and brief illness duration (less than 3 years); (2) patients with a young age of onset but longer duration of illness; and (3) patients with an older age of onset (i.e., after 19 years of age). Treatment lasted 1 year, and sessions were typically conducted a weekly intervals. Over the 5 years of the study, four therapists treated most of the patients, each taking on both individual and family therapy cases. Outcome was evaluated at 1-year follow-up. Overall, the results were not encouraging; only 13 of the anorectics (23%) had a good outcome, while 34 (60%) had a poor outcome. Family therapy was significantly more helpful for the subgroup that has an early age of onset and short duration, whereas for the other two subgroups as well as for the bulimic anorectics, the results of family therapy were not different from those of individual therapy. The study thus found family therapy to be more effective than individual therapy in young, nonchronic anorectic patients.

Group Therapy and Support Groups

Very little has been written about group therapy for anorectics. Hall (1985) discussed in some detail the difficulties of group therapy for anorectics, namely, the patients' rigidity, withdrawal, high anxiety and dysphoria, outward compliance, hypersensitivity to criticism, constant preoccupation with weight and food, difficulty in identifying and expressing feelings, tendency to escape from disturbed thoughts and feelings or situations by losing weight, and competitiveness with one another. All these characteristics tend to inhibit self-disclosure, sharing and confrontation, making it difficult to foster a spirit of camaraderie or group identity. Other therapists have relied on more experiential and nonverbal techniques to specifically address such issues (e.g., Crisp et al., 1985; Wooley & Wooley, 1985), but the results have not been documented. It may also be worthwhile to try with anorectics the more structured and psychoeducational approach employed with bulimics (Mitchell, Hatsukami, Goff, Pyle, Eckert, & Davis, 1985). As it stands, group therapy relying more on experiential techniques should probably be used as an adjunctive treatment for anorectics to decrease isolation and withdrawal. It is perhaps not advisable to mix males with females or bulimics with anorectics, since such combinations may further increase competitiveness and inhibit sharing.

Support groups generally consist of patients at various stages of treatment and recovery as well as their families. In contrast to self-help groups, support groups always encourage the patient to seek professional treatment. The groups are usually led by a recovered patient and/or a parent of a patient, although sometimes professionals are also involved in a supportive capacity. The greatest benefit lies in giving information and peer support and in confronting reluctant or resistant patients to encourage them to begin or continue treatment. There is some concern among clinicians that thrusting patients prematurely into a helping role may result in their deriving vicarious satisfaction from helping others instead of dealing with their own personal issues. In general, if the groups are led by experienced facilitators, then the benefits usually outweigh the disadvantages.

Psychoeducational Treatment

Since many anorectic patients are still in their school years, the fact that hospitalization may take several months mandates the presence of psychoeducational support within the hospital. A special education teacher who works in close liaison with the school should therefore be assigned to the eating disorders unit. Anorectics are usually over-achievers, and some limits may have to be set on how much time they can spend on schoolwork. Vocational guidance may be necessary for the older teenager who is unsure about career changes and opportunities. Expressive arts therapy using drama, music, or painting, conducted either individually or in a group, may be helpful, particularly when the patient has difficulty in verbalizing feelings. The techniques described by Wooley and Wooley (1985), already reviewed, may be used.

Pharmacotherapy

In the past 30 years many medications have been used for the purpose of inducing weight gain (Crisp, 1965; Dally & Sargant, 1960), correcting the hypothesized central neurotransmitter dysfunction (Marrazzi & Luby, 1986; Needleman & Waber, 1977; Vigersky & Loriaux, 1977), or allaying patients' anxiety about eating (Andersen, 1987; Crisp et al., 1985). Chlorpromazine (a neuroleptic) was widely used initially to reduce anxiety and resistance by promoting sedation. However, it has significant side effects, including hypotension, hypothermia, and grand mal seizures, and its efficacy has never been formally tested. Vandereycken (1984) and Vandereycken and Pierloot (1982) found sulpiride and pimozide (other forms of neuroleptics) marginally better than placebo, but the crossover design and other methodological limitations in their studies, which we will comment on later, made interpretation of the results difficult. More recently, Vandereycken

(1987) has concluded that neuroleptics are of minimal benefit in the treatment of anorexia nervosa. Antidepressants were apparently effective in inducing weight gain in several open trials (Mills, 1976; Needleman & Waber, 1977), but in a double-blind study of amitriptyline, cyproheptadine, and placebo in 72 anorectic inpatients in an 8-week study (Halmi, Eckert, LaDu, & Cohen, 1986), the effect of amitriptyline (a tricyclic antidepressant) on weight gain and depressed mood was at best marginal. In this large-scale study, 23 patients were randomized to amitriptyline, 24 to cyproheptadine, and 25 to placebo. Amitriptyline produced a significantly more rapid weight gain measured in terms of days needed to reach target weight. However, the proportion of patients receiving placebo who eventually reached target weight was not different from that of patients receiving amitriptyline. In addition, the antidepressant effect of amitriptyline was not clearly superior to placebo. Furthermore, it did not improve anorectic attitudes and behaviors. A controlled study using clomipramine (another tricyclic antidepressant) did not find it to have any effect on weight or mood (Lacey & Crisp, 1980). Cyproheptadine, an antiserotonin and antihistamine drug, produced conflicting results in two earlier double-blind studies (Goldberg, Halmi, Eckert, Casper, & Davis, 1979; Vigersky & Loriaux, 1977), and in the recent 8-week trial on 72 anorectic inpatients already mentioned (Halmi et al., 1986), its effect on weight gain and mood change was marginal. The patients receiving cyproheptadine had a more rapid weight gain when compared with those on placebo, but the rate of weight gain was not different from that of patients on amitriptyline. Again, cyproheptadine was not more effective than placebo in inducing a larger proportion of patients to achieve target weight. Cyproheptadine produced a significant improvement in mood by day 14, and this effect may have persisted to day 28, but this is unclear from the data presented. It did not improve the patient's self-ratings on eating attitudes and behaviors. On a measure called "treatment efficiency," cyproheptadine was better than placebo for the restrictive anorectics and worse for the bulimic anorectics. Lithium carbonate, in an 8-week inpatient trial, apparently induced more rapid weight gain than placebo (Gross et al., 1981). Findings of the double-blind studies are summarized in Table 6.1. Thus existing evidence suggests that some psychotropic medications may have a marginal effect on the rate of weight gain in an anorectic patient when used in conjunction with behavioral or milieu treatment.

Defining what constitutes meaningful improvement in anorexia nervosa is a major difficulty that investigators must grapple with. All the medication studies have used rate of weight gain as an index of improvement, and I have already stated that it is pointless to do so. Rapid weight gain is uncomfortable and possibly dangerous to the patient and bears no relationship to long-term outcome. Furthermore, since competent inpatient care by itself can bring 85% of patients to their target weights, it may be difficult to prove that medications confer any additional benefit. A more meaningful approach may be to study whether medication can prevent relapse after the patient has regained a healthy weight. Unfortunately, no studies have evaluated the effect of medication on relapse prevention or long-term outcome.

Treatment of Concomitant Psychiatric Symptoms

Depression is common in anorexia nervosa, but it is rarely severe and in general it improves with weight gain (Eckert et al., 1982; Halmi et al., 1986; Morgan & Russell, 1975). Its content is always related to a fear of fatness or loss of control (Crisp, 1980; Hsu, 1980). As already mentioned, it may also respond to antidepressants and cyproheptadine. However, unless a patient meets the criteria for major depression, the indications for use of these medications are unclear. Most clinicians probably treat the depression as a part of the anorectic illness, but Morgan and colleagues (1983) found it necessary to use antidepressant in 60% of their patients at an unspecified dosage. Social anxiety, obsessive–compulsive features (Crisp, Hsu, & Harding, 1980; Morgan & Russell, 1975), and sexual fears (Beumont, Abraham, & Simson, 1981; Crisp, 1980) are also common, and they may not improve with weight gain (Cantwell et al., 1977; Hsu & Crisp, 1980; Morgan & Russell, 1975). However, they are usually viewed as a part of the anorectic disorder and treated with individual psychotherapy; to my knowledge, specific treatments have not been studied. Schizoaffective symptoms, sometimes brief in duration, may develop in the context of the anorectic illness, but they appear to run a course separate and distinct from the eating disorder (Grounds, 1982; Hsu, Meltzer, & Crisp, 1981). However, they may also occur after apparent recovery from the anorectic illness and persist into schizophrenia. Neuroleptics and antidepressants are probably the

TABLE 6.1. Controlled Medication Studies of Anorexia Nervosa

Study	Duration	Design	N	Dose	Effect of drug and placebo on rate of weight gain	Other effects
Antidepressants						
Clomipramine Lacey & Crisp (1980)	≤ 4 months	Parallel group	16	50 mg/day	None	Drug increased hunger, appetite, and energy
Lithium carbonate Gross et al. (1981)	4 weeks	Parallel group	16	Therapeutic plasma level	Drug better	Conflicting results
Amitriptyline Halmi et al. (1986)	≤ 3 months	Parallel group, drug vs. placebo and cyproheptadine	72	≤ 160 mg/day	Drug better	Drug may reduce depression; no effect on eating attitude
Cyproheptadine						
Vigersky & Loriaux (1977)	8 weeks	Parallel group	24	≤ 12 mg/day	None	None
Goldberg et al. (1979)	5 weeks	Parallel group, with and without behavior therapy	81	≤ 32 mg/day	Drug better in severely ill subgroup with birth complications	None

Halmi et al. (1986).	≤ 3 months	Parallel group, drug vs. placebo and cyproheptadine	72	≤ 32 mg/day	Drug better	Drug may reduce depression; no effect on eating attitude
Neuroleptics						
Pimozide Vandereycken & Pierloot (1982)	3 weeks	Crossover	18	≤ 6 mg/day	None	None
Sulpiride Vandereycken (1984)	3 weeks	Crossover	18	≤ 400 mg/day	None	Drug produced better scores than placebo on the Eating Attitudes Test

treatment of choice and are usually effective in controlling such symptoms.

Outpatient Treatment

As already mentioned, less emaciated patients who are not vomiting, purging, or suicidal may be treated as outpatients. The treatment goals, already stated, are also valid for this poulation, but it is unclear how much emphasis should be placed on weight gain, since positive reinforcement or nursing care is difficult to implement in an outpatient setting. The clinician who wants to tackle the weight issue will therefore have to rely heavily on nutritional education, which should be given along the lines already described. In addition, regular weighing should probably be implemented, if only to make certain that the patient does not drop below a minimum agreed-upon weight. As an alternative to nutritional counseling, some therapists make an agreement with the patient that outpatient therapy will be discontinued if she drops below a certain weight (e.g., Orbach 1985). In effect, this puts the responsibility of maintaining a minimum weight on the patient. Dare (1983), in the context of outpatient family therapy, asks the family to take the responsibility of making the patient eat and gain weight, and the preliminary results seem encouraging. As already mentioned, this approach may be more applicable to the younger patient (Russell et al., 1987). Coercive treatments are obviously not applicable for the outpatient. The indication for antidepressants in the absence of depression is unclear, but they do not in general seem to induce weight gain and, if the patient suspects that they would, she will usually resist taking them.

The mainstay of outpatient treatment for anorexia nervosa is therefore psychotherapy aimed at resolving the underlying psychological problems. Individual and family psychotherapy along the lines already described should therefore be implemented. Adjunctive treatment, such as group therapy or social-skills training, may also be given. Patients who respond to outpatient psychotherapy by gaining weight seem to do better in the long term (Hsu, Crisp, & Harding, 1979; Morgan et al., 1983), although they may be less ill to begin with.

Relapse after inpatient treatment is common (Hsu et al., 1979; Russell et al., 1987), occurring perhaps in at least 50% of patients within the first year of discharge. Outpatient therapy should therefore always follow inpatient treatment. Treating an anorectic patient who dutifully returns to each session and yet loses exactly 1 pound a week can be a harrowing experience. Prevention of relapse is thus one of the most difficult treatment tasks, but unfortunately very little research has been conducted in this area. However, the clinician should remain cautiously optimistic since experience indicates that although most patients will lose some weight upon discharge from the hospital, many will regain it with continued outpatient care. Again, a combination of individual, family, nutritional, and perhaps group therapy form the mainstay of treatment. Russell (1970, 1977b) suggests repeated hospitalizations until the patient grows out of her illness.

Treating the Bulimic Anorectic Patient

The bulimic anorectic patient is at special risk for developing hypokalemia and cardiac arrest (Halmi, 1978; Isner, Roberts, Heymsfield, & Yager, 1985; Russell, 1979), and the cessation of vomiting and laxative and diuretic abuse on admission to the hospital may precipitate abrupt fluid retention and rapid weight gain (MacGregor, Markandu, Roulston, Jones, & de Wardener, 1979). Inpatient treatment may temporarily break the vicious cycle of binge-eating and vomiting, but the bulimic behavior, while clearly related to "a starved body demanding to be fed" (Russell, 1979, p. 447), unfortunately does not always cease with weight gain (Hsu, 1980). For the normal-weight bulimic patient, both cognitive therapy and antidepressants have proven to be effective (see section "Treating Bulimia Nervosa"), but their efficacy for the bulimic anorectic patient has apparently not been evaluated. Cooper and Fairburn (1984) have reported encouraging results in a preliminary study in which cognitive therapy was used. Family therapy was not more effective than individual supportive therapy in the Maudsley study that we have already reviewed (Russell et al., 1987).

Treating Chronic Patients

About 30% of patients remain ill 4 to 10 years after the onset of illness (Chapter 7), and Dally (1969) has suggested that a patient who has been continuously ill for more than 7 years is unlikely to respond to treatment. The long-term outcome of these patients is unfavorable, although for many years they may function relatively well at a stable but low body weight. Aggressive treatment of a chronic patient may precipitate depression or even suicide (Crisp, 1980), and thus the clinician should carefully review the treatment goals for each patient. Perhaps the best approach is to encourage some weight gain that will not take the patient to the population average. A paradoxical approach may occasionally be useful. In a preliminary study of eight patients, Hsu and Lieberman (1982) told the patients that since they had held on to their anorexia nervosa despite various attempts to cure it, then they must perceive the illness to be of great personal significance and value. They further suggested that the patients should therefore retain their anorexia nervosa but at the same time to try to understand its unique value and significance. At 2 and 4 year follow-up, half of the patients had regained their normal weight. Antidepressants (in particular the newer ones such as fluoxetine) may be given if depressive symptoms occur and may be helpful in alleviating such symptoms, although in my experience they do not alter the anorectic attitude and behavior. Electroconvulsive treatment and leucotomy are rarely, if ever, helpful. Great clinical acumen and skills are needed in the management of such patients. Fortunately, a clinician dealing mainly with adolescent patients will not see many chronic cases.

Nevertheless, it is my experience that one should retain hope even in a most recalcitrant case. The following case illustrates how empathic understanding, flexibility, perseverance, and therapeutic skills can bring about recovery even in a seemingly hopeless situation:

> A 39-year-old woman had developed bulimic anorexia nervosa at the age of 17. In the subsequent 20 years, her weight fluctuated between 35 kg and 50 kg; she had not been able to refrain from bingeing and vomiting for longer than a few weeks; and she had at various times abused alcohol, laxatives, tranquilizers, and diet pills. She had had several lengthy periods of inpatient treatment at a renowned eating disorder clinic but could not maintain her improvement. She had made several suicide attempts, usually in relation to altercations with her father, a domineering naval commander, or her husband (30 years her senior) whom she had married much against her father's wishes at the age of 27. At age 36 her weight had again dropped to 35 kg (height, 164 cm), and she was bingeing and vomiting several times a day, and abusing alcohol and tranquilizers. She refused

the offer to be readmitted to the eating disorders clinic because she could not accept the target weight set at 52 kg. She became very depressed, took yet another overdose, and was treated in two inpatient units without success.

A psychiatrist in private practice agreed to take her on for twice-a-week individual psychotherapy provided she could maintain her weight above 35 kg. She gradually improved and at the last follow-up had maintained her weight at 48 kg for 1 year, and had not binged; vomited; or abused laxatives, alcohol, tranquilizers, or diet pills for 18 months. She was eating three meals a day, and her menses had returned for the first time in 20 years. She ascribed her improvement to "being understood" by her psychiatrist, and to having the opportunity to discuss her fears and conflicts without pressure to gain weight. It is also important to note that within this psychotherapeutic relationship she was able to implement, without further specific help, what she had previously learned about healthy eating habits in the eating disorders clinic.

TREATING BULIMIA NERVOSA

By the time a bulimic patient presents for evaluation at the clinic, she is generally more motivated for treatment because she finds the symptoms to be distressing. However, she may want to control her binge-eating simply so she can lose weight and thus may be disappointed when she realizes that weight loss is not the primary goal of treatment. Moreover, bulimic patients are sometimes very impulsive, and if the symptoms do not resolve quickly, they are liable to become discouraged. Nevertheless, in the 10 years since the disorder has been separated from anorexia nervosa, clinicians have made some progress in its treatment. The following discussion focuses on treating the normal-weight bulimic, since treatment of the bulimic anorectic has just been described. Treating the overweight bulimic is discussed in a separate section toward the end of the chapter.

Treatment Goals and Treatment Setting

The first treatment goal is to establish a regular eating pattern and eliminate the binge–purge–starve cycle. The second treatment goal is to change the thoughts, beliefs, and feelings that perpetuate the bulimic behavior. The third goal is to treat the physical complications and concomitant psychiatric symptoms that are common in bulimia nervosa. Finally, since the course of the illness is sometimes character-ized by periods of remission and exacerbation, the fourth treatment goal is to prevent relapse. Again, while most clinicians will find these treatment goals valid, there are some who perceive the eating distur-bance to be a secondary phenomenon and thus prefer to work with the patient on deeper psychodynamic or personality issues. Of course, as a matter of strategy, the therapist may choose to focus on issues other than the eating behavior at different times during the course of treatment. However, it is the distinct experience of many clinicians (e.g., Fairburn, 1985; Mitchell, Hatsukami, Goff, Pyle, Eckert, & Davis, 1985) that unless the eating problems are tackled directly, they do not as a rule improve, even when the underlying issues are resolved.

Most bulimic patients can be treated successfully as outpa-tients. Indications for inpatient admission are the presence of serious physical complications, suicidal ideation or behavior, and failure of outpatient treatment.

In practice the first two treatment goals are usually tackled by a combination of nutritional and cognitive–behavioral treatments. For the sake of clarity and because they are conceptually distinct, the two treatments will be discussed separately.

Dietary Treatment

While the exact etiology of bulimia nervosa is unknown, there is evidence to suggest that it is related to strict and prolonged dieting and that a pattern of regular eating may ameliorate the bulimic behavior. Clinically, most patients have reported that the bulimia was preceded by a period of dieting to lose weight (Cooper & Fairburn, 1983; Pyle, Mitchell, & Eckert, 1981). Perhaps 50% of bulimic patients have a previous history of anorexia nervosa (Hsu & Holder, 1986; Lacey, 1983). Even when they refrain from bingeing or purging, bulimic patients show a highly abnormal eating pattern: 80% of bulimic patients eat one meal or less a day (Hsu, in press; Mitchell, Hatsukami, Eckert, & Pyle, 1985). Most patients starve themselves during the day only to give in to the overpowering urge to binge in the evening. In experimental situations, chronic dieters ("restrained eaters") would overeat once they perceived that they had violated their dietary control (Polivy, Herman, Olmsted, & Jazwinski, 1984). This is consistent with the bulimics' experience that eating may trigger a binge, particularly if they eat food they normally forbid themselves (i.e., "blow their diet"). While researchers have not clearly established that individuals who habitually diet and occasionally binge will eventually develop bulimia nervosa, there is clearly an overlap between subclinical bulimia and pathological bulimia nervosa (Patton, 1988b; Szmukler et al., 1985; Yager, Landsverk, & Edelstein, 1987). Finally, the Minnesota Experiment conducted more than 40 years ago (described in some detail at the beginning of Chapter 2) demonstrated clearly that semistarvation may lead directly to extreme overeating, even in healthy non-weight-preoccupied young men (Keys et al., 1950). The finding that, after refeeding, some of the men became very concerned about the tendency of fat to accumulate in the abdomen and buttocks was particularly intriguing (Keys et al., 1950, p. 828). While these men did not develop an eating disorder per se, the evidence is compelling that chronic starvation could lead to dramatic changes in eating behavior and mental state, many of which closely resemble those that occur in diagnosable anorexia and bulimia nervosa.

Given the association between self-imposed starvation and binge-eating, it is surprising that so little attention has been given to dietary treatment in bulimia nervosa. Most treatment programs for bulimia nervosa include a dietary treatment component, but it is rarely described separately and specifically and its efficacy has not been independently assessed. Many studies included meal planning and nutritional education as a part of their treatment (Hsu & Holder, 1986; Huon & Brown 1985; Johnson, Schlundt, & Jarrell, 1986; Kirkley, Schneider, Agras, & Bachman, 1985; Roy-Bryne, Lee-Benner, & Yager, 1984; Wolchik, Weiss, & Katzman, 1986) but gave no details. A few studies (Fairburn, 1981; Hsu & Holder, 1986; Lacey, 1983) used weekly monitoring of body weight. Kirkley and colleagues (1985) compared two different group treatments, one of which used some aspects of what could be called nutritional counseling, such as instructing the patients to eat regular meals, increase the variety of foods eaten, decrease the eating rate, and eat forbidden foods in a nonbinge setting. Although this approach was significantly more effective than the nondirective approach, it was impossible to ascribe the improvement to the nutritional counseling, since this was combined with instructions to delay vomiting and to use relaxation training tapes.

Dietary treatment for bulimia nervosa is aimed at educating the patient in the principles of good nutrition, assessing personal nutritional needs, explaining the relationship between starvation and overeating, and making clear the effects of vomiting and purging. In addition, it is aimed at helping the patient plan balanced meals each day and develop a healthy eating pattern. Some clinicians may include the establishment of a healthy exercise pattern as an additional goal.

The principles of dietary treatment for the bulimic patient are therefore similar to those for the anorectic. However, while an anorectic is asked to gain weight, the bulimic is usually asked to maintain her weight at presentation (e.g., Hsu & Holder, 1986; Mitchell, Hatsukami, Goff, Pyle, Eckert, & Davis, 1985). Garner, Rockert, Olmsted, Johnson, & Coscina (1985) recommend that the goal weight be within a range of about 5 pounds (about 2.5 kilograms) of 90% of the patient's highest weight prior to the onset of her eating disorder, although for some patients they also recommend that they should let their weight settle at a level that does not require chronic dieting to maintain. I use the latter approach. The dietician may initially calculate the patient's caloric requirements based on the need for about 30 kilocalories/kilogram/day or may consult a food nomogram (e.g., Pemberton & Gastineau, 1981). Subsequent requirements may be adjusted according to actual intake and weight change. Some clinicians advise against calorie counting (e.g., Fairburn, 1985), and in practice it is probably best to use one's judgment about whether the patient will become too obsessed with it. It is, however, essential that the patient know enough about nutritional requirements and the nutritional content of foods to be able to plan three to four meals a day, each containing balanced amounts of carbohydrates, protein, and fats, as well as fruits and vegetables. Several meetings with a dietician may be required.

The reluctance of many patients to follow such a meal plan should be anticipated, since they are usually concerned that they will gain weight. The dietician should then explain the effects of starvation, the relationship between starvation and binge-eating, and the ineffectiveness of purging to control body weight. Further, the dietician should explain that some weight fluctuation is normal at this stage, since rebound fluid retention may occur with decrease in the bingeing and purging, and that body weight will eventually stabilize with improvement. Again, the clinician should be reminded that despite their avid interest in food and dieting, many bulimics harbor distorted and mistaken notions about them; hence, detailed discussions on these topics are essential.

Initially it is probably advisable for the patient to avoid foods that lead to a binge (e.g., Mitchell, Hatsukami, Goff, Pyle, Eckert, & Davis, 1985). With improvement, it may be helpful for the patient to eat small amounts of binge foods in nonbinge settings. I will return to this point in the section below on Stage Two. Since some patients experience anxiety in eating with others or eating in a restaurant, a few sessions of eating in a restaurant with a dietician or a nurse may be useful. Finally, some patients complain that when they enter a supermarket, they instinctively go for the binge foods. Thus some practice sessions with a dietician or a nurse in supermarket shopping with prior planning of what to purchase may be helpful.

Cognitive–Behavioral Treatment

Cognitive–behavioral treatment arises out of the conceptualization that bulimia nervosa occurs as a set of dysfunctional behaviors that represent "a difficulty in coping with disturbed feelings and thoughts" (Fairburn, 1982, p. 631). Binge-eating has been interpreted as a response to stress (Pyle et al., 1981), a means of modulating dysphoric or anxiety states (Loro & Orleans, 1981), a behavior to meet an unfulfilled emotional need (Russell, 1979), a way of controlling her weight when she fails to control other events in her environment (Hawkins & Clement, 1980), or a release from the control she has imposed upon herself in her striving to be perfect (Boskind-Lodahl, 1976). These interpretations on the meaning of the bulimic behavior are consistent with the patient's self-report that the urge to binge is often triggered by such emotional states as dysphoria, anger, tension and boredom and that overeating, particularly of fattening, "forbidden" foods, initially produces a sense of satisfaction, nurturance, oblivion, or liberation, although this is soon followed by a sense of defeat and guilt (see Chapter 2). Some researchers have emphasized the primary role of vomiting or purging as a maladaptive means of relieving the anxiety associated with eating (Rosen & Leitenberg, 1982), but most patients insist that they engage in such behaviors only to get rid of the calories. Many, however, enjoy the fact that they can eat whatever they want without gaining weight, and a few find the purging to have a relaxing or "cleansing" effect. Johnson and Connors (1987) have stated in summary that the bulimic behavior may serve to regulate affect, express oppositionality and impulsivity, and function as a means of self-nurturance. Finally, many female patients relate their chronic dysphoria and frustration to their low self-acceptance and self-worth, a constant need to appear slim, and a fear of negative evaluation and rejection, particularly from men. These experiences have led researchers, such as Boskind-Lodahl (1976) and Orbach (1985), to postulate that bulimia nervosa is related to the complex and conflicting role of women in Western society.

The primary aim of cognitive–behavioral treatment is to change the cognitions preceding a binge, counter the bulimic behavior, and improve the patient's poor self-acceptance. The assumption is that these elements perpetuate the patient's bulimic behavior.

Garner, Fairburn, and Davis (1987) recently reviewed 19 studies of acceptable methodology published between 1981 and 1986. While the studies differed in the details of their design, by and large they attempted to evaluate the effectiveness of various cognitive–behavioral techniques. The following review draws on the common elements of all these studies.

Treatment may most conveniently be divided into three stages (Fairburn, 1985), although this is not always explicitly stated in the studies.

Stage One

The aims of the first stage of treatment are to disrupt the binge–purge–starve cycle, to introduce a pattern of regular eating, and to provide information regarding the relationship between starvation and binge-eating and the potentially dangerous consequences of purging. It is also common to begin to explore the functions of the bulimic behavior at this stage.

The therapist therefore relies heavily on a psychoeducational approach. However, the success or failure of treatment sometimes hinges on whether a positive therapeutic relationship can be built at this stage. The therapist should therefore be supportive and encouraging and should try to anticipate the patient's difficulties so that plans can be made with the patient to counter them. At the same time, the therapist should be firm and authoritative when necessary, particularly when it comes to insisting that the patient eat regular meals and monitor her daily intake.

If possible, the therapist should enlist the help of an experienced dietician to assist the patient in planning three to four meals a day. If this is not possible, the therapist should gain enough nutritional knowledge to suggest a balanced meal plan. Some patients may initially be very resistant to eating three or four meals a day, and at this stage it may be preferable to suggest that they eat at least two meals a day. The greatest concern of the patient is that she will gain weight and become obese if she eats meals. Several approaches may be beneficial: explanation and reassurance, teaching the patient to anticipate some weight fluctuation due to the rebound fluid retention that occurs with a decrease in bingeing and purging, and attendance at a support group where recovered bulimics share their experiences. The patient may also find it helpful to read an article, such as "Psychoeducational Principles in the Treatment of Bulimia and Anorexia Nervosa" (Garner, Rockert, Olmsted, Johnson, & Coscina, 1985), that explains the basic principles of diet and weight.

Some simple stimulus-control techniques may be helpful at this stage. Patients should be asked to eat slowly, to limit eating to a specific setting only, to eschew other activities (e.g., watching television) while eating, to limit the food available when eating, and to avoid storing any binge foods in the home. In addition, the dietician or therapist may help the patient plan her shopping list and schedule so that she does not impulsively buy binge foods once she goes shopping.

A major treatment task at this stage is to help the patient monitor her eating. All the cognitive–behavioral studies regard this as an essential step in the patient's gaining control over her eating behavior. Self-monitoring increases the patient's awareness of her eating pattern in general and her bulimic behavior in particular. It helps both her and the therapist understand her eating pattern, the antecedents of binges, and the frequency and timing of the bulimic episodes. Such an understanding allows the patient and the therapist to devise techniques to combat the binges and purges. Patients should be asked to record their food and liquid intake immediately after its consumption and to indicate whether they were consumed as part of a meal, a snack, and/or a binge. The patient may initially find it difficult and embarrassing to write down everything she eats or drinks, and this should be anticipated and discussed in detail. It is essential that the intake charts be reviewed and analyzed at each session. Methods of improving monitoring should be discussed at each session, and accurate monitoring should be praised.

After a few sessions the patient and therapist can usually identify the antecedents to binges. These events may be physiological (e.g., hunger or tiredness), emotional (e.g., anger, dysphoria, boredom, anxiety, or frustration), cognitive (e.g., feeling fat or unattractive, or the thought that "now that I've blown it I might as well go on bingeing"), or situational (e.g., being alone, getting critical comments from mother or boyfriend, being invited to a party). Similar antecedents may precede the self-induced vomiting or taking of laxatives. Patients are sometimes relieved to see that there is, after all, a "reason" for their binge-and-purge behavior.

Different programs vary in terms of their timing and emphasis on abstinence from binge eating. Some make no specific mention of it (e.g., Fairburn, Kirk, O'Connor, & Cooper, 1986), others expect immediate abstinence (e.g., Mitchell, Hatsukami, Goff, Pyle, Eckert, & Davis, 1985), and yet others anticipate a gradual reduction in the frequency of episodes (e.g., Hsu & Holder, 1986). It is unclear which approach is more effective, although Mitchell, Hatsukami, Goff, Pyle, Eckert, and Davis (1985) found the expectation of immediate abstinence to work best in their experience. The intensity of treatment will be discussed later, but, in general, it would appear that severely ill patients may do better with high-intensity treatment (two or more sessions a week) to begin with, while less severely ill patients may do well with weekly sessions.

Stage Two

After the patient has been able to adhere to a regular pattern of eating and to decrease the episodes significantly (at least 75%), she may feel ready to move on to the second stage of treatment. The aims of the second stage are to maintain a pattern of regular eating, to reduce the excessive dietary restrictions, to continue to identify the antecedents for the bulimic episodes, to develop ways to combat such antecedents and reduce their frequency, and to counter the specific fear of fatness. Most therapists tackle the binges, assuming that when the binges cease, so will the purges. Others directly seek to eliminate the self-induced vomiting and to reduce the anxiety associated with eating (e.g., Ordman & Kirschenbaum, 1985; Wilson, Rossiter, Kleifeld, & Lindholm, 1986).

Monitoring of eating behavior should continue at this stage, and deviation from a regular pattern should be discussed. The clear expectation is that the patient should maintain a regular pattern of eating. While during the early stages of treatment it is usually advisable to ask the patient to avoid binge foods, at the second stage of treatment her excessive dietary restrictions should be tackled. As already mentioned, patients often divide foods into good and bad categories based on mistaken notions, and the bad foods are usually high-carbohydrate and high-fat foods that she craves but forbids herself. The sight and tasting of such foods may trigger a binge. The patient initially gives in to the craving and, once the first bite is taken, has the feeling that all is lost (i.e., she is going to get fat) and that she might as well go all the way and make the most of her failure, since she can always vomit afterwards. To tackle this problem, the patient may either be asked to eat a small amount of binge food in a nonbinge setting outside of the treatment session (where loss of control is unlikely to occur), or to bring a small amount of the binge food to one or more sessions and eat it in the presence of the therapist, a technique discussed at the end of this section. The patient should also be encouraged to incorporate a wider variety of foods into her meals, and a dietician may be helpful here. Admittedly, a small number of patients may prefer to follow a model of total abstinence, banishing all binge foods, such as those containing white sugar, from their diet. It is unclear how successful this approach is in the long run.

A variety of cognitive–behavioral techniques are used to counter the antecedents to the bulimic episodes. Broadly speaking, they fall into two major categories: problem-solving techniques and modification or restructuring of dysfunctional cognitions that perpetuate the bulimic behavior. Both approaches rely heavily on the cognitive therapies of Beck (1976), Ellis (1962), and Meichenbaum (1977; for review of these therapies, see Hollon & Beck, 1986). Fairburn (1985) has described in detail a seven-step model for problem solving: defining the problem, identifying alternative solutions to the problem, identifying the implications of each solution, choosing one solution, defining the steps to implement the solution, executing the solution, and evaluating the entire problem-solving process. The problems that bother the bulimic patient usually involve interpersonal issues. For instance, to be asked out to dinner is a problem on several levels: what to wear, whether to eat beforehand, how interested the male friend is in her, whether her mother will approve, and so forth. These questions are always related to the patient's thoughts, beliefs, and, ultimately, values, many of which are distorted and dysfunctional. The identification and modification or restructuring of such thoughts and beliefs are therefore essential to treatment. The therapist should engage the patient in Socratic discussion; after identifying a dysfunctional thought (e.g., "I am fat"), the arguments in favor of it as well as against it should be examined in order to reach a reasoned conclusion (Fairburn, 1985). For each thought the patient should ask herself: "Is it true? What is the evidence for or against it? If true, what does it mean? What might be the other alternative explanations for my thought or perception? What are the consequencs of my thought or perception? What are the advantages and disadvantages of holding onto this thought or perception? What options do I have in dealing with it?" (Chester, 1989). Garner, Rockert, Olmsted, Johnson, and Coscina (1985) described various techniques of cognitive restructuring for the eating-disorder patient: techniques such as decatastrophizing ("What if the feared solution really happened?"), decentering ("Do people really notice that my stomach is bloated?"), challenging the patient's "shoulds" ("Should I always do what is expected, should I always be perfect"), and reattribution ("I feel fat because I have an eating disorder"). Other dysfunctional cognitions (McKay, Davis, & Fanning, 1981) that should be restructured include: mind reading ("Everyone thinks I am unattractive"), emotional reasoning ("I feel fat, therefore I am fat"), polarized thinking ("I am not perfect therefore I am a failure"), and global labeling ("I have gained one pound therefore I am a failure"). In between sessions, the patient is given self-instructional exercises based on these techniques to counter the desire to binge or to purge, to problem solve, and to modify her moment-to-moment dysfunctional thoughts and cognitions. At each session the difficulties surrounding a particular situation are discussed in detail (e.g., going home to visit parents), using a cognitive–behavioral approach.

The patient's characteristic fear of fatness may be dealt with by cognitive restructuring. As already mentioned, Wooley and Wooley (1985) have used experiential techniques to tackle this body-image distortion. Other themes, such as the sociocultural pressure on women to be thin and the conflicting roles of women in contemporary society (Boskind-Lodahl, 1976; Orbach, 1985), are also introduced for discussion at this stage of treatment.

Various therapists (e.g., Ordman & Kirshenbaum, 1985; Rosen & Leitenberg, 1982, 1985; Wilson et al., 1986) have also focused on preventing vomiting after the patient has eaten binge foods. This approach, commonly called "exposure and response prevention," is based on an anxiety-reduction model: Vomiting reduces the anxiety of eating, which in turn is associated with the fear of being fat. The therapist asks the patient to bring to the session a small amount of binge food and to eat it in the therapist's presence to such a point that she feels uncomfortable and wants to vomit ("exposure"). The therapist then engages the patient in a variety of therapeutic tasks and discussions, such as cognitive restructuring, until her discomfort and desire to vomit diminish and disappear ("response prevention"). After a few sessions the patient may practice the technique at home.

Stage Three

The goals of stage three are to prepare the patient for termination and to discuss relapse prevention.

Termination is discussed in the usual way, confronting the patient's feelings of loss and uncertainty. Relapse prevention is important, since apparently a substantial number of successfully treated patients suffer temporary relapses. The patient should be informed that relapses may occur at times of stress or when she attempts to diet to lose weight. She should be told that monitoring of food intake, which is generally phased out at stage three, should be resumed if she feels her eating is out of control. The patient should also be instructed to practice the self-instructions she has learned to counter the urges to binge or starve, to solve problems, and to modify her dysfunctional cognitions. If significant improvement does not occur in a matter of a few weeks, the patient should be encouraged to contact the clinic again. Finally, after overcoming their eating disorder some patients may want further, more psychodynamic, treatment to deal with their personal issues. Appropriate referrals should be made at this stage.

Duration, Intensity, and Format of Treatment

Published treatment studies vary in terms of their duration of treatment, the frequency of their sessions, and whether the treatment was conducted individually, in a group, or in a combination of both. Some treatments last a few weeks (e.g., Lee & Rush, 1986), while others may last much longer (e.g., Fairburn, 1981; Roy-Bryne et al., 1984). It is unclear at this stage what the optimal duration of treatment is. Giles, Young, and Young (1985) found that some patients who fail to respond to brief treatment may respond to longer, more protracted treatment. If a patient fails to improve significantly after a few weeks of cognitive therapy, it is my practice to consider the use of medication (see section on Practical Suggestions, below).

In most of the studies, sessions were conducted once a week, although some began with twice-weekly sessions (e.g., Fairburn et al., 1986). Mitchell, Hatsukami, Goff, Pyle, Eckert, and Davis (1985) started the patients with five sessions a week in various group formats, such as lectures and formal group therapy discussions, and then tapered to twice a week at the end of 8 weeks of treatment. It seems logical that a severely ill patient may do better with a higher frequency and intensity of treatment, while a less severely ill patient may do quite well on once-a-week sessions.

Some treatments were conducted in groups (e.g., Dixon & Kie-colt-Glaser, 1984; Huon & Brown, 1985; Schneider & Agras, 1985), some were conducted individually (e.g., Fairburn et al., 1986; Hsu & Holder, 1986), and some used a combination of group and individual treatments (e.g., Lacey, 1983; Wolchick et al., 1986). The relative effectiveness of group versus individual treatment has not been studied. In their review, Garner, Fairburn, and Davis (1987) indicate that group therapy may be associated with a higher dropout rate. Clearly some patients prefer the camaraderie of a group and the support that patients can give to one another, while others prefer the more individual attention of a therapist and find the self-disclosure in a group setting uncomfortable. The choice of treatment depends on the preference of both patient and therapist.

Treatment Results

In the 19 studies reviewed by Garner and colleagues (1987) there was on average a 79% reduction in binge frequency from pre- to post-treatment, with a range of 51% to 97%. At the end of treatment, which lasted a few weeks to a year, between 20% and 80% of the patients were no longer bingeing or vomiting. To the best of my knowledge, eight controlled studies have been published (Fairburn et al., 1986; Freeman, Sinclair, Turnbull, & Annadale, 1985; Kirkley et al., 1985; Lacey, 1983; Lee & Rush, 1986; Ordman & Kirschenbaum, 1985; Russell et al., 1987; Wilson et al., 1986). Their findings and design are summarized in Table 6.2, which also summarizes the findings of a ninth study (Wolchik et al., 1986) that was not strictly speaking a controlled study, since patients were not randomly allocated to the treatment conditions. All those that used a waiting-list group as a control condition found active treatment to be vastly superior (Lacey, 1983; Lee & Rush, 1986; Ordman & Kirschenbaum, 1985). Cognitive treatment was somewhat more effective than short-term therapy (Fairburn et al., 1986) and nondirective therapy (Kirkley et al., 1985). Exposure and vomit prevention, when used in conjunction with cognitive restructuring, was more effective than the latter alone (Wilson et al., 1986). In sum, all these studies indicate that cognitive–behavioral treatment, even for a relatively brief period, is effective in the control of bulimic behavior, at least in the short term.

However, among all 19 of these studies some have clearly superior results (e.g., Fairburn et al., 1986; Freeman et al., 1985; Kirkley et al., 1985; Lacey, 1983) when compared to others (e.g., Hsu & Holder, 1986; Lee & Rush, 1986; Wilson et al., 1986). There is no immediate explanation for such discrepancies, since the patient populations and the techniques used were essentially similar (Wilson et al., 1986). Perhaps the problem lies with the assessment of bingeing and purging. All the studies relied on patient self-report of binge-and-purge behavior as the principal outcome measure, but the reliability and validity of this measure is subject to many factors, such as the patient's definition of what constitutes a binge and the accuracy of the recall (Garner, Fairburn, & Davis, 1987). Rosen and Lietenberg (1982) and Ordman and Kirschenbaum (1985) recommended exposing the patient to a standardized test meal and measuring the amount of food consumed as well as grading the discomfort and urge to binge afterwards. This may provide a more objective outcome measure. Others (see section in Chapter 2 entitled "Experiential Aspects") are exploring the possibility of measuring the patient's eating behavior in a controlled environment for a period of up to 24 hours. Until some objective measure is available and used by all studies, the problem of why some investigators are more effective than others may never be answered.

TABLE 6.2. Controlled Psychotherapy Studies for Bulimia

Author/treatment	Diagnostic criteria	N	Individual/ group/family	Duration of treatment	% reduction in B/V pre- to post-treatment
Fairburn et al. (1986)	Russell			18 weeks	
Cognitive–behavioral		12	I		88/93
Focal (i.e., insight & cognitive)		12	I		82/87
Freeman et al. (1985)	DSM-III			15 weeks	
Cognitive (+ minimal behavioral)		15	I		94/—
Behavioral (+ minimal cognitive)		15	I		92/—
Group (? nature)		15	G		96/—
Waiting list		15	—		0 (?)/—
Kirkley et al. (1985)	DSM-III-R equivalent			16 weeks	
Cognitive–behavioral		14	G		97/95
Nondirective		14	G		64/70
Lacey (1983)	Russell			10 weeks	
Cognitive–behavioral + insight		15	I & G		95/96
Waiting list		15	—		0/0
Lee & Rush (1986)	DSM-III			6 weeks	
Cognitive–behavioral		15	G		70/69
Waiting list		15	—		0/13
Ordman & Kirschenbaum (1985)	DSM-III			4-22 weeks	
Cognitive–behavior + E & RP[a]		10	I		—/78
Brief (i.e., waiting list)		10	—		—/30

Study / Treatment	Diagnosis	N		Duration	Outcome
Russell et al. (1987)	Russell			1 year	No difference between family & individual treatment (see text)
Family therapy		9	F		
Individual insight + supportive		10	I		
Wilson et al (1986)	DSM-III equivalent			16 weeks	
Cognitive–behavioral		9	G		51/58
Cognitive–behavioral + E & RP[a]		8	G		83/89
Wolchik et al. (1986)	DSM-III			7 weeks	
Cognitive–behavioral		11	G		58/53
Waiting list (nonrandom)		7	—		69/79

[a]Exposure and response prevention

Family Therapy

Relatively little has been written regarding family therapy for bulimia nervosa patients. Since bulimic patients are usually older and thus no longer living at home, family therapy may be less feasible. They are perhaps also more ashamed of their behavior and thus reluctant to involve the family. Family issues are therefore more commonly dealt with in individual or group therapies. Investigators have found a variety of characteristics in the families of bulimic patients (e.g., Root, Fallon, Friedrich, 1986; Schwartz, Barrett, & Saba, 1985). However, it is extremely unlikely that the various family pathologies that have been described are peculiar to the bulimic family. Nevertheless, the bulimic patient is often at the developmental stage of separating from her family, and individuation issues may need to be worked through. Separation difficulties are often compounded by the patient's tendency to be outwardly compliant and yet jealous and competitive. These patients will therefore need family therapy, or at least individual therapy dealing with family issues. In a controlled study comparing family therapy with individual supportive therapy in 23 bulimia nervosa patients, Russell and colleagues (1987) found neither to be particularly effective. It may be that their patients were suffering not from normal-weight bulimia nervosa but from bulimic anorexia nervosa, which may be particularly resistant to treatment (e.g., Hsu, 1980). However, it may also be that their treatments were relatively ineffective because they were not focused directly on the aberrant eating behavior. Either way, their finding would indicate that family therapy as a primary treatment for bulimia nervosa may not be particularly effective.

Pharmacotherapy

There is good evidence to indicate that antidepressants are effective in the short-term treatment of bulimia nervosa. Evidence for the efficacy of anticonvulsants and other pharmacological agents is more meager.

Antidepressants

The use of antidepressants in bulimia nervosa probably arises from the observation that the disorder may be associated with an affective illness (see Chapter 4). Early uncontrolled studies found monoamine oxidase inhibitors (Rich, 1978; Walsh, Stewart, Wright, Harrison, Roose, & Glassman, 1982) and tricyclic antidepressants (Pope & Hudson, 1982) to be effective in controlling the binge-eating.

To the best of my knowledge, there are to date six double-blind controlled studies using antidepressants (these, as well as two studies discussed in the below section on Other Psychotropic Medications, are summarized in Table 6.3). One used a tetracyclic, four a tricyclic, and one a monoamine oxidase inhibitor (MAOI). The British study (Johnson-Sabine, Yonace, Farrington, Barrett, & Wakeling, 1983) used mianserin, a tetracyclic antidepressant not marketed in this country, because of its relative lack of side effects. A total of 50 female, normal-weight bulimic outpatients were randomly allocated to 60 mg of mianserin or placebo for 8 weeks. Presumably the patients were seen at weekly intervals for medication management, but it is unclear whether other treatments, if any, were given concurrently. In the end, 30 were on placebo and 20 on mianserin, but 14 (6 on drug, 8 on placebo) out of the 50 patients did not complete the study. Mood and eating attitudes improved significantly for both groups, but bulimic behavior did not change in either group. Because the study was characterized by a high dropout rate, the findings are difficult to interpret. It is also doubtful if 60 mg of mianserin was sufficient to constitute a therapeutic dosage for all the patients. Blood levels of mianserin were taken, but the findings have so far not been reported.

Pope and colleagues (1983) used imipramine (200 mg) and placebo in a 6-week double-blind trial of 22 female, normal-weight bulimic outpatients. Overall, the imipramine group had a 70% decrease in binge frequency and 50% decrease in depression rating, whereas the placebo group was virtually unchanged on both measures. Only 3 patients dropped out (2 on drug, 1 on placebo). The patients did not receive any other form of supportive treatment during the study. Mitchell and Groat (1984) randomized 32 female bulimic outpatients to amitriptyline (150 mg) or placebo for 8 weeks. The subjects also received a minimal behavioral treatment program, which consisted of advice to eat three meals a day and not to worry about their weight, daily self-monitoring of eating behavior, and verbal reinforcement by the physician for improvement in eating behavior. Six patients dropped out of the study (5 on drug, 1 on placebo). In both groups there was a significant improvement in

TABLE 6.3. Controlled Pharmacotherapy Studies for Bulimia

Author	Treatment	N	Diagnostic criteria	Duration	Outcome
Agras et al. (1987)	Imipramine/placebo	10/10	DSM-III	16 weeks	Imipramine significantly reduced purging at 6 and 16 weeks, significantly reduced depression at 6 but not 16 weeks
Hsu et al. (undated)	Lithium carbonate	Depressed, 11/7; nondepressed 27/23	DSM-III-R equivalent	8 weeks	Lithium better in decreasing bingeing and purging for depressed bulimics; no difference in other variables; both lithium and placebo nondepressed patients improved significantly
Hughes et al. (1986)	Desipramine/placebo	11/11	DSM-III	6 weeks	Desipramine significantly reduced episodes, abnormal eating attitudes, and depression
Mitchell & Groat (1984)	Amitriptyline/placebo	16/16	DSM-III	8 weeks	No difference between drug and placebo on episodes; drug significantly reduced depression
Pope et al. (1983)	Imipramine/placebo	11/11	DSM-III-R equivalent	6 weeks	Imipramine significantly reduced episodes and depression

Johnson-Sabine et al. (1983)	Mianserin/placebo	20/30	Russell	8 weeks	High dropout from both groups; no difference between drug and placebo on episodes
Walsh et al. (1984)	Phenelzine/placebo	13/13	DSM-III	8 weeks (after 2 weeks of placebo washout)	Phenelzine significantly reduced episodes, abnormal eating attitudes, and depression
Wermuth et al. (1977)	Phenytoin/placebo crossover	10/10	DSM-III equivalent	6 weeks, then 6 weeks crossover	Phenytoin significantly reduced episodes but carryover effect was present

eating behavior, while the amitriptyline group improved significantly more on one measure of depression. Depressed bulimics did less well than the nondepressed, whether on drug or placebo. Serum drug levels were available for 8 subjects on the active medication; those who had attained a therapeutic level had a better response.

Hughes, Wells, Cunningham, and Ilstrup (1986) randomized 22 nondepressed, female bulimic outpatients to desipramine (200 mg) and placebo in a 6-week trial. Apart from weekly visits, apparently no other supportive treatment was given. Patients on desipramine had a 91% decrease in binge frequency, while those on placebo had a 19% increase. At the end of the study, the patients on placebo were given desipramine and the dosage in all patients was adjusted according to their blood level. In the event, 15 of the 22 patients achieved abstinence from binge-eating.

Agras, Dorian, Kirkley, Arnow, and Bachman (1987) randomized 20 female bulimic outpatients to either imipramine (up to 300 mg) or placebo for 16 weeks. Patients on the active medication had a significantly greater decrease in their purge episodes at both week 6 and week 16 than those taking placebo. Data on binge episodes were, however, not reported. There was a significantly greater decrease in the depression scores at week 6 for those on imipramine, but this advantage over those on placebo was no longer present at week 16. Behavioral techniques were specifically avoided during the weekly sessions.

Walsh and colleagues (1984) randomized 35 bulimic female outpatients to phenelzine (an MAOI) and placebo for 8 weeks. Only 20 patients completed the study (9 on drug, 11 on placebo). The high dropout occurred in part because the authors used a 2-week placebo washout period, thereby excluding the placebo responders, and in part because phenelzine produced significant side effects leading to early termination. Five of the 9 patients on phenelzine ceased bingeing completely, none on placebo did so, and only 2 on placebo decreased their episodes by more than 50%. Apparently no concurrent supportive treatment was given.

Recently fluoxetine (Prozac) has been studied in a large, multicenter, 8-week trial for bulimia nervosa (Enas, Pope, & Levine, 1989). Treatment at 60 mg is apparently associated with significant improvement in binge-and-purge episodes, but details of the study are not available at the time of this writing.

In summary, antidepressants are effective for bulimia nervosa when given in a therapeutic amount. Independent of an antidepressant effect, 60% to 70% of patients have experienced a significant reduction in number of binge-and-purge episodes. It is unclear at this point which antidepressant is the most effective. It is also unclear how long a patient should be maintained on an antidepressant to achieve long-term remission.

Other Psychotropic Medications

In 1974 Green and Rau treated ten patients with compulsive over-eating with Dilantin in an open trial. Nine ceased to binge-eat with the medication. The authors believed that the patients' episodic ego-dystonic overeating had certain epileptic-like features. In a subsequent larger open trial, Rau and Green (1984) reported that 70% of 38 bulimic patients with abnormal EEGs improved significantly in terms of a decrease in binge-eating, while 35% of those without abnormal EEGs improved similarly. However, these studies were uncontrolled, and many clinicians may take issue with the authors' observations and theoretical underpinnings. Their observation that the binges occurred without reason is particularly disturbing, since their patients were apparently all dieting to lose weight. Wermuth, Davis, Hollister, and Stunkard (1977) randomized 20 female bulimic outpatients to a 12-week crossover study of phenytoin (at least 300 mg/day) versus placebo. In both the drug–placebo and placebo–drug sequence, phenytoin was significantly more effective than placebo in reducing binge frequency. However, the results were difficult to interpret because the crossover design allowed for a carryover effect of improvement. Experience suggests that patients who improve will maintain their improvement for at least a short while, and thus a crossover design may not be appropriate for medication studies of bulimia nervosa. Further, the authors included obese as well as emaciated subjects in their study, and this heterogeneity in patient population most probably confounded their findings. Unfortunately no other controlled study using phenytoin has been published.

Kaplan (1987b) in a crossover double-blind study using carbamazepine and placebo, found that the active medication did not overall have a significant antibulimic effect on the 16 bulimic patients studied.

Fenfluramine, a serotonergic agonist marketed as an appetite suppressant, significantly decreased intake in a laboratory setting in bulimic patients 2 hours after it was given in a single, oral, dose of 60 mg (Robinson, Checkley, & Russell, 1985). Two double-blind treatment trials found conflicting results. Russell, Checkley, Feldman, and Eisler (1988) in a 12-week trial of 42 outpatients found only a suggestion of benefit of the medication, and primarily among those who dropped out of the study. However, the high dropout rate (17/42) could have affected the results of the study. Blouin and colleagues (1988) in a crossover design of two 6-week periods with a 3 week washout period in between, found fenfluramine to be at least as effective as desipramine in significantly decreasing binge-and-purge episodes in 22 patients. Both desipramine and fenfluramine also significantly improved the patients' depressed mood.

Hsu, Clement, Santhouse, Deep, and Ju (undated) divided 91 female bulimic outpatients into two groups, depressed and nondepressed, and separately randomized them to take either lithium carbonate (up to 1200 mg/day) and placebo for 8 weeks. Sixty-eight patients completed the study. Overall, nondepressed patients improved equally and significantly not only in terms of their binge episodes but also in terms of their psychopathology as measured by a variety of instruments. Lithium had a greater benefit over placebo for those who were depressed, since the depressed/placebo group was the only one not to show a significant decrease in their binge/purge episodes from pre- to post-treatment.

Inpatient Treatment

It is my experience as well as that of others (e.g., Mitchell, Hatsukami, Goff, Pyle, Eckert, & Davis, 1985) that probably 10% of bulimic patients require inpatient treatment. Inpatient admission is indicated for the very depressed or suicidal patient so that intensive treatment can focus on both the depression and the bulimic disorder. The presence of severe physical complications is another indication, but for this a patient may be admitted to a general medical or surgical ward. Patients who fail to improve with outpatient treatment may be able to break their bulimic cycle with the external control and intensive treatment available on an inpatient unit. For this reason, admission of the patient to a specialized eating-disorder unit is probably preferable than admission to a general psychiatric ward, where such specialized supervison and treatment may not be available.

Treatment of Bulimia in Obese Subjects

Obese individuals sometimes binge-eat, and such episodes are followed by severe discomfort and feelings of self-condemnation (Stunkard, 1959). Recent studies suggest that about 25% of obese patients report serious problems with binge-eating (Gormally, Black, Daston, & Rardin, 1982; Loro & Orleans, 1981). These patients usually do well on weight-loss programs, since they can successfully follow the strict dietary constraints of such programs. Unfortunately, they can almost never maintain the weight loss because of the binge-eating, and the treatment of binge-eating in the obese is a major clinical issue (Gormally, 1984). At this stage it is unclear whether bulimia is a homogeneous disorder for individuals at different weight levels. As already mentioned, the *DSM-III-R* gives no weight criteria for the diagnosis of bulimia nervosa. Although self-induced vomiting or purging is rare among the obese, the subjective experience of a binge episode appears to be similar whether the subject is overweight, of normal weight, or underweight.

In my view, clinicians must first decide whether to treat the obesity or the binge-eating. Weight reduction and cessation of bulimia are not identical or interchangeable goals. It is possible that in some individuals the two goals may actually be incompatible. The association of starvation and binge-eating has already been discussed. Unfortunately, studies that focus on the treatment of bulimia in obese subjects are rare, and those that exist include both normal-weight and obese binge-eaters in their samples (e.g., Hawkins & Clement, 1980). Clearly all the treatment principles described above for bulimia nervosa may be applicable for bulimia in the obese. Their efficacy, however, has yet to be determined.

PRACTICAL RECOMMENDATIONS

For anorexia nervosa, I usually recommend inpatient treatment in the first instance. Nursing care and nutritional treatment combined with psychotherapy form the mainstay of treatment, although behavioral principles, such as positive reinforcement and information feedback, are used as well. Social-skills training, expressive arts therapy, and other nonverbal therapies are also instituted for the inpatients. Long-term eclectic individual psychotherapy is given after the patient's discharge. For an adolescent patient, family therapy is almost always used for both the inpatient and outpatient. Medication is used only when definitely indicated; that is, if depressive or psychotic symptoms exist. However, some flexibility is necessary in treating chronic patients.

It is my practice to begin treatment of normal-weight bulimia nervosa with individual cognitive–behavioral therapy, conducted at weekly or twice-weekly intervals. Patients are also encouraged to attend a weekly support group, either at the clinic or elsewhere locally. If there is no improvement after 4 weeks, then treatment with a tricyclic antidepressant is instituted, and the blood level of the medication is monitored. A tricyclic antidepressant is preferable to a monoamine oxidase inhibitor, because the side effects are usually more benign and a rigid diet is not required. Family therapy is given if significant family issues exist, and family members are also invited to attend a support group. Subsequently, patients who improve significantly on individual treatment may be asked to join a 10-week structured psychoeducational group. In the weekly group meetings, a staff member begins by giving a fifteen-minute lecture on a topic relevant to the group, such as one of those suggested by Weiss, Katzman, and Wolchik (1985). This is followed by a group discussion and review of homework assignments, which include self-monitoring of food intake. If the tricyclics cause intolerable side effects or are ineffective, we substitute them with fluoxetine, beginning with 20 mg in the morning and gradually increasing the dosage at three-week intervals (a gradual increase is preferable in my view because of the long half-life of fluoxetine). Blood fluoxetine level is monitored. If a patient is not significantly better after three or four months, then inpatient treatment is recommended.

Sometimes patients have had extensive psychotherapy before they come to the clinic. If they have not already had medication, then I begin treatment with a tricyclic antidepressant. If a tricyclic has been used and found ineffective, I may use either an MAOI, such as tranylcypromine, or fluoxetine. It is important to remember that a medication-free period of 2 weeks should be instituted before substituting an MAOI for a tricyclic (or vice versa) or when substituting one MAOI for another (such as changing from tranylcypromine to phenelzine). A 5- to 6-week medication-free period should be instituted when substituting fluoxetine for an MAOI or vice versa. It is our experience that medications should always be used with supportive psychotherapy.

CASE ILLUSTRATION

Pam, the 17-year-old high school junior whose presentation and history were described in Chapter 5, began treatment in our clinic by meeting with a registered dietician, who prescribed 1,500 calories a day divided into three meals and one evening snack. About 50% of the calories were to be in the form of carbohydrates and 25% each, protein and fat. Pam was taught the exchange system, and each day she was to eat about nine bread exchanges, two milk exchanges, five meat exchanges, five fat exchanges, and three exchanges each of vegetables and fruits. Cognitive therapy consisted of meeting with the psychiatrist each week. She had to record the circumstances of her eating, particularly the events that preceded a binge, as well as her food intake each day. Plans to combat the urges to binge and vomit were devised at each meeting following a careful review of her dietary-monitoring sheets. In addition, the psychiatrist explained in detail the relative inefficacy of diet pills and their potential dangers, and he strongly discouraged her from using them. After 8 weeks of treatment, Pam was able to successfully overcome all urges to binge, although she still had difficulty combating urges to vomit. She discontinued her diet pills for 5 consecutive weeks, but in the eighth week took four caffeine pills.

After 8 weeks of treatment, Pam's eating disorder was largely under control, and the psychotherapy therefore centered more on

adolescent issues in general rather than on the eating disorder itself.
She was also seen on a number of occasions with her mother to discuss
their relationship, particularly the overinvolvement of the mother in
Pam's life. A female therapist took over from the psychiatrist and
conducted both the individual and the mother–daughter sessions
from this point onwards. After 6 months Pam was bingeing and
vomiting very sporadically (about once or twice every 2 months on
average) and had discontinued the use of diet pills. She was then asked
to join a weekly psychoeducational group for bulimic patients, which
ran for 10 weeks. Topics such as fear of fatness, proper nutrition and
effects of starvation, assertiveness, depression and anxiety, parents,
boyfriends, and the role of women were systematically covered in
these sessions, which were jointly led by a nurse and a social worker.

As summer vacation approached, the family moved to their
summer house, and Pam was not seen for 2 months. The mother
entered her into a beauty contest, but despite the pressures to be slim,
Pam did not revert to vomiting or abusing diet pills. However, when
the new school year began, Pam became more depressed and anxious,
and the binge-and-vomit episodes increased to about once or twice a
week. Individual weekly sessions with the same therapist were resumed.
It was decided at this point that a trial of an antidepressant might be
worthwhile, and she was therefore given desipramine up to a dose of
150 mg/day. After 6 weeks she regained control over her bulimic
behavior, and the desipramine was discontinued after 6 months.

Pam then enrolled in an out-of-state college, and so treatment
was formally terminated. Just before she was due to leave home, the
father was taken to the hospital because of a sudden deterioration in his
physical health. The physician informed him and the family that his
liver function was quite impaired because of his alcoholism and strongly
urged him to seek treatment, which he again declined. The mother
decided to leave the father and moved out of the house. Despite the
stress, Pam did not revert to her bulimic behavior, and she managed to
leave home to attend college. Telephone contact 2 years after termination of treatment indicated that she remains symptom-free.

Assessment Results

These were presented in Table 5.6. After 8 weeks of treatment there
was an obvious improvement in the bulimic behavior and the EDI

and EAT scores. The BDI and SCL-90 scores, normal to begin with, dropped further. However, SAD and FNE scores did not change. At 1-year follow-up improvement in the eating behavior and EDI and EAT scores were maintained. The BDI and SCL-90 scores were normal. Again, there was no change in SAD and FNE scores, which remained abnormally elevated.

Comment

As already mentioned in the text, individual cognitive–behavioral and nutritional treatment can often be quite successful. It is gratifying to note that Pam's improvement was maintained despite continuing parental problems. The persistently high SAD and FNE scores perhaps indicated Pam's overconcern for the approval of others, and this perhaps led to the increased anxiety and depression at the beginning of her senior year in high school.

7

Outcome

The outcome of anorexia nervosa has been a subject of considerable debate among investigators, although more recently some agreement has been reached regarding its intermediate term (4- to 12-year) outcome. The prognosis for bulimia nervosa is yet to be determined, because the illness has only recently been separated diagnostically from anorexia nervosa and only a few outcome studies have been conducted.

Knowledge of the outcome of a disorder is important for at least the following reasons. It will prevent us from confusing short-term improvement with long-term cure. It will allow us to evaluate our treatment efforts and, more specifically, how they fare against the natural course of the illness. It may help us identify the prognostic indicators, which in turn may allow us to better anticipate what course the illness may take. It may help settle the debate over the identity and nosology of the eating disorders. I discuss here all these issues in the context of a review of the outcome of the eating disorders.

OUTCOME OF ANOREXIA NERVOSA

In 1954, Beck and Brochner-Mortensen undertook one of the earliest outcome studies on anorexia nervosa. They were prompted to do so after a debate on the topic among internists and psychiatrists during a case conference at the Copenhagen University Hospital. Opinion has always differed widely on the outcome of anorexia nervosa. Gull (1874) regarded it as for the most part favorable, and Hurst (1939) stated that "a few straight forward conversations are sufficient" (p. 745) to straighten out the mental tangles of an anorectic. However, German psychiatrists such as Meyer (1961) and Cremerius (1965) had emphasized the likelihood of chronicity in many patients. In reviewing 16 major studies published between 1954 and 1979, I (Hsu, 1980) came to the conclusion that, overall, 75% of patients had improved at follow-up 4 to 8 years later, 20% had become chronic, and about 5% had died from the illness. A subsequent review of 45 studies by Steinhausen and Glanville in 1983 did not seem to contradict these findings.

Nevertheless, there are wide variations in outcome among individual studies. Some have claimed that the better outcome in some studies is due directly to better treatment (e.g., Minuchin et al., 1978; Thoma, 1967). Others have suggested that, since very few patients remained anorectic at follow-up but many had instead developed an affective disorder, anorexia nervosa may in fact be an affective illness (e.g., Cantwell et al., 1977). Before these claims can be accepted, it may be helpful to examine some of the methodological defects that could account for the discrepant findings among the studies:

1. *Lack of a rigorous definition of the syndrome.* This failing characterized many of the earlier studies. For instance, Bliss and Branch (1960) defined anorexia nervosa as a state of nervous malnutrition and included in their series all patients with a weight loss of more than 25%, whatever the psychological cause. Seidensticker and Tzagournis (1968) included patients without amenorrhea, while 29% of patients in Silverman's study (1977) had a diagnosis of schizophrenia. Whatever one's view regarding the identity of the disorder, it is imperative that in an outcome study the criteria of diagnosis be stated explicitly.

2. *Failure to use a direct method of follow-up.* Denial of illness among anorectics is common. Indirect methods of follow-up, such as the use of questionnaires and telephone interviews, thus run the risk of yielding inaccurate information and failing to detect minor morbidity. Many studies failed to report on the exact method of follow-up (e.g., Rosman et al., 1977), while others used predominantly indirect

methods of interview (e.g., Cantwell et al., 1977; Garfinkel, Moldofsky, & Garner, 1977).

3. *Failure to trace patients.* A high failure-to-trace rate affects the results of any outcome study. In anorexia nervosa the effects may be further compounded by the fact that patients who are still ill are less likely to cooperate. For instance, both Cantwell and colleagues (1977) and Thoma (1967) failed to trace some 20% of their patients. It is therefore very likely that they might have missed those patients who were still anorectic.

4. *Short duration of follow-up.* Cycles of recovery and relapse are common in anorexia nervosa, and several studies have shown that successful weight gain during inpatient treatment did not result in long-term cure (Hsu et al., 1979; Morgan & Russell, 1975). Therefore, the illness may not have run its full course if outcome is measured over an insufficiently long period (Russell, 1970). Those studies that focused on patients with a short follow-up duration (e.g., Rosman et al., 1977) are likely to yield biased results.

5. *Inadequate outcome criteria.* Many authors have used only one outcome measure (e.g., Lesser et al., 1960). This is inadequate, since improvement in one area does not necessarily reflect improvement in others. Furthermore, because many studies did not define what was meant by "normal," "cured," or "recovered," the findings are difficult to interpret. For instance, Cantwell and colleagues (1977) rated only one patient (5% of total sample) as having possible anorexia nervosa at follow-up, but elsewhere Sturzenberger, Cantwell, Burroughs, Salkin, and Green (1977) reported that body-weight outcome in the same series was poor in some 20% of the patients. Such contradictions are hard to reconcile. Several patients in Beck and Brochner-Mortensen's series (1954) were rated as recovered, but their body weight was below 80% of average. If these patients were rated as not recovered, as they should have been, then the authors' optimistic conclusions might not be tenable. Rosman and colleagues (1977) did not define what they considered to be normal weight. Needless to say, such failings can lead to serious confusion.

6. *Incomplete information at follow-up.* Since emaciation and amenorrhea are the cardinal features of anorexia nervosa, it is surprising that many outcome studies failed to report on body weight and menstrual status at follow-up (e.g., Bruch, 1973; Halmi, Brodland, & Loney, 1973; Valanne, Taipale, Larkio-Miettinen, Moren, & Aukee,

1972; Williams, 1958). These failings are particularly puzzling because such information can be gathered and evaluated quite easily without much subjective bias (Russell, 1970, 1977b). Many studies failed to report on patients' eating behavior at follow-up, perhaps on the unfounded assumption that restoration of body weight goes hand in hand with normalization of eating behavior. Finally, information on the patients' mental status and psychosocial functioning were often sketchy.

Recent Outcome Studies

Recently, five studies that used essentially the same methodology and outcome criteria have been published (Burns & Crisp, 1984; Hall, Slim, Hawker, & Salmond, 1984; Hsu et al., 1979; Morgan et al., 1983; Morgan & Russell, 1975). These studies, which are summarized in Table 7.1, shared the following characteristics:

1. All the studies used explicitly stated diagnostic criteria such that atypical cases were excluded. Morgan and colleagues (1983) and Morgan and Russell (1975) used Russell's criteria (1970); Burns and Crisp (1984) and Hsu and colleagues (1979) used Crisp's criteria (1977); while Hall and colleagues (1984) used the Washington University criteria (Feighner et al., 1972). Despite these differences, from the demographic and weight characteristics reported we can conclude that all the patients in the five series had anorexia nervosa with similar severity.

2. All the studies followed the patients for at least 4 years. Morgan and Russell (1975) dated the duration of their follow-up from hospital discharge; Burns and Crisp (1984), Hsu and colleagues (1979), and Morgan and colleagues (1983) dated their studies from time of presentation; and Hall and colleagues (1984) dated the duration of follow-up from the onset of illness. Despite these differences, the duration from onset of illness for all the series is probably similar, although the series of Burns and Crisp (1984) and Hall and colleagues (1984) may have contained more patients with a shorter duration of illness. The onset of illness is sometimes hard to define, depending on whether it is dated from the onset of dieting, major weight loss, or amenorrhea; because many patients have received only outpatient treatment and because discharge from inpatient care does not mean

TABLE 7.1. Overview of Follow-up Studies in Anorexia Nervosa

Study	Total no. of cases/sex/ no. of inpatients	N (total) traced	Duration	Method
Burns & Crisp (1984)	27/M/20 IP	27 (100)	2–20 years after evaluation	Personal interview with 23 (85%)
Hall et al. (1984)	50/F/36 IP	49 (98)	4–12 years after onset of illness	Personal interview with 43 (86%)
Hsu et al. (1979)	105/F/49 IP	102 (97)	4–8 years after evaluation	Personal interview with 75 (75%)
Morgan et al. (1983)	73/F/5/M/41 IP	75 (96)	4–8 years after evaluation	Personal interview with 69 (88%)
Morgan & Russell (1975)	38/F/3/M/all IP	41 (100)	4–10 years after discharge	Personal interview with 34 (79%)

treatment termination, it may be preferable in future studies to date the follow-up duration from the time of presentation to the investigators' clinic. All five of the studies are best described as intermediate-term outcome studies, a point I will return to later.

3. All the studies had a low failure-to-trace rate (less than 5%) and a high direct-interview rate (more than 70%). Thus the findings are less likely to be biased.

4. All the studies used multiple and well-defined outcome criteria. As already mentioned, confusion can easily arise if only global outcome scores are used or if the outcome ratings are undefined. All five studies used Morgan and Russell's (1975) outcome criteria, and direct comparison of their findings is thus possible.

However, these studies still had certain methodological flaws. None used a standardized structured or semistructured interview for assessment of patients' mental state at follow-up. Very few standardized self-report measures were used. None of the studies specifically addressed the question of the relationship between anorexia nervosa and affective illness or anorexia nervosa and bulimia nervosa; however, this shortcoming is understandable, since interest in these issues is more recent. The duration of follow-up in all the studies was relatively brief. At the time of follow-up, which occurred at 4 to 12 years after the onset of illness, the patients would have been in their late 20s or 30s, at which time the illness might not have run its full course. Finally, none of the studies expressed mortality in terms of standardized mortality ratio, thus making it impossible to compare mortality rates between studies or with age- and sex-specific mortality rates of the general population.

Other recent studies that attempted to overcome such methodological deficiencies unfortunately had other failings. For instance, the Toronto group has recently published a 5- to 14-year follow-up of a consecutive series of 149 anorexia nervosa patients seen between 1970 and 1978 at the Clark Institute (Toner, Garfinkel, & Garner, 1986). Standardized interviews and self-report measures were used in the assessment of outcome. The authors also included a control group of nonanorectic women for comparison. Unfortunately, the failure-to-trace rate was high: Only 74 of the 149 patients were located for follow-up, and of these 14 decided not to participate in the study. Thus the final sample consisted of 60 patients; 55 were interviewed and 5 were dead at the time of the follow-up. The high failure-to-trace rate, in my view, seriously impairs the validity of the findings.

Overall Outcome

Given their methodological similarities, it is perhaps not surprising that outcome in the five studies was very similar (see Tables 7.2 and 7.3). Between 50% and 60% of patients were at normal weight, and 47% to 58% were having regular menses. Between 11% and 20% of the patients were still markedly underweight at follow-up. It is perhaps remarkable that the outcome in males was essentially the same as that in females. Theander's earlier study (Theander, 1970), which used similar weight and menstrual-status criteria, also found 51% at outcome to have a normal body weight and 66% to have regular menses.

However, an improvement in weight does not necessarily indicate a normalization of eating attitudes and behavior (see Table 7.4). All the studies found that two out of three patients at follow-up were still intensely preoccupied with weight and dieting and that a regular eating pattern occurred only in about one-third of the patients. As discussed later, bulimia nervosa, not major depression, is probably the most common diagnosis after anorexia nervosa at follow-up. However, these findings are not based on the use of standardized measures, and none of the studies used a control group.

Mortality

The five studies showed a crude mortality rate of 0% to 5% for anorexia nervosa. Unfortunately, none of the studies presented the results in terms of standardized mortality ratio. Emaciation and suicide were the most common causes of death. Patton (1988a), in a 4- to 15-year follow-up study of 460 eating-disorder patients (332 anorectics, 96 normal-weight bulimics, and 32 with other eating disorders), found a 600% increase in the mortality of anorectics when compared with the expected ratio in the general population and a 940% increase for bulimics. There were no deaths among those—subclinical anorectics and bulimics—categorized as having other eating disorders. For the anorectics, most of the deaths occurred within the first 8 years after initial consultation, particularly within the first 4. This finding is

TABLE 7.2. Mortality, Weight, & Menstruation at Follow-Up

Author	Mortality	Normal	Weight over	Very low	Menstrual outcome regular	Amenorrhea
Burns & Crisp (1984)	0%	52%	4%	11%	Not applicable	
Hall et al. (1984)	1%	50%	10%	14%	50%	32%
Hsu et al. (1979)	2%	62%	2%	15%	51%	28%
Morgan et al. (1983)	1%	At least 58%	—	—	At least 58%	At least 19%
Morgan & Russell (1975)	5%	55%	5%	20%	47%	39%

TABLE 7.3. Outcome (Percent of Patients) According to Morgan's
Outcome Category

Author	Good	Intermediate	Poor	Death	Untraced
Burns & Crisp (1984)	44	26	30	0	0
Hall et al. (1984)	36	36	24	2	2
Hsu et al. (1979)	45	30	20	2	3
Morgan et al. (1983)	58	19	19	1	3
Morgan & Russell (1975)	39	27	29	5	0
Mean	44	28	24	2	2

consistent with Theander's (1985) long-term study, which is described below in the section on Long-Term Outcome of Anorexia Nervosa. More than one previous admission and a lower weight at presentation predicted a fatal outcome for anorexia nervosa. Six of the eleven deaths among the anorectics occurred as a result of suicide, while emaciation was most likely the cause of death for the other 5. The proportion of bulimic anorectics ($n = 25$, 8%) was uncharacteristically low among the entire cohort of anorectics, and, unexpectedly, none died from their illness. However, one of the bulimics died as a result of developing anorexia nervosa (see section on Mortality under Outcome of Bulimia Nervosa, below). The high standard mortality ratio of anorexia nervosa is clearly a subject of great concern.

Mental Status Outcome

As already mentioned, one of the major shortcomings among the five studies was their failure to use a standardized interview for the assessment of mental state at outcome. Morgan and Russell (1975) found 45% to show affective (usually depressive) symptoms and 23%, obsessive symptoms. It is unclear how many would have qualified for a diagnosis of an actual disorder. Hsu and colleagues (1979) found 38% and 22% to report depressive and obsessive symptoms, respectively, but again it is unclear how many would qualify for a "case" of major depression or obsessive–compulsive disorder. One patient was diagnosed as having bipolar disorder, and three had schizophrenia. Burns

TABLE 7.4. Eating Difficulties at Follow-Up

Author[a]	Preoccupation with wt/food	Normal eating	Dieting	Bulimia	Vomiting	Purgative	Anxiety eating with others
Burns & Crisp (1984)	63%	37%	—	7%	11%	11%	26%
Hall et al. (1984)	62%	—	—	40%	26%	—	—
Hsu et al. (1979)	72%	35%	46%	19%	21%	34%	31%
Morgan & Russell (1975)	63%	33%	50%	—	25%	33%	51%

[a]Morgan et al. (1983) did not describe eating difficulties at follow-up.

and Crisp (1984) found eight patients (30%) to have marked psychiatric disturbances; of these, three (11%) were alcohol or substance abusers, one (4%) had severe obsessive neurosis, and four (15%) displayed unspecified disorders. In addition, six (22%) had mixed phobic anxiety and depressive symptoms. Hall and colleagues (1984), using the *DSM-III* criteria for diagnosis, found 34% to have a dysthymic disorder, 6% to have major depression, 4% to be alcohol abusers, and 2% each to have schizophrenia, bipolar disorder, and personality disorder. In total, a significant proportion of patients (perhaps one-third) at follow-up had at least quite significant depressive symptoms, and perhaps about 10% would have qualified for major depression. However, all the studies indicated that the affective symptoms occurred predominantly in the context of significant eating-disorder symptoms; that is, patients who remained anorectic were more likely to suffer from concomitant affective symptoms. As already mentioned, the Toronto group (Toner et al., 1986) used a standardized interview schedule (Diagnostic Interview Schedule, Version III) for the assessment of patients' mental status. For a lifetime diagnosis, 61.5% of the restrictive anorectics met criteria for an affective disorder, 57.7% for an anxiety disorder, 23.1% for a substance use disorder, and 3.8% for a somatization disorder, while 52.4% of the bulimic anorectics met criteria for affective disorder, 66.7% for anxiety disorder, 42.9% for substance use disorder, 4.8% for somatization disorder, and, finally, 4.8% for schizophrenic disorder. These figures were significantly higher than those found in the control group of nonanorectic women. Within the last year of the interview, 38.4% of the restrictive anorectics met criteria for affective disorder, 42.3% for anxiety disorder, 3.8% for somatization disorder, while 28.5% of the bulimic anorectics met criteria for affective disorder, 52.4% for anxiety disorder, 42.9% for substance use disorder, 4.8% for somatization disorder, and 4.8% for schizophrenic disorder. Again, these figures were significantly higher than those found in the control group. Differences between the restrictive and bulimic anorectics for both lifetime and past-year diagnosis were not significant, except that bulimic anorectics had a significantly higher prevalence of substance use disorder. Unfortunately, the researchers did not state whether the patients who qualified for a concurrent psychiatric diagnosis were still anorectic or bulimic.

Psychosexual and Psychosocial Outcome

Without adequate control data, the findings on psychosexual outcome are difficult to interpret. The proportion of women who were married at follow-up varied from 28% (Hsu et al., 1979) to 40% (Hall et al. 1984). Thirty percent of the males in the Burns and Crisp series (1984) were married at follow-up. Obviously, factors other than psychiatric ones affect the institution of marriage in a given society. Abnormal sexual attitudes (fear or disgust toward sex) occurred in 20% (Hsu et al., 1979) to 37% (Burns & Crisp, 1984) of the patients, but the findings were not based on standardized interviews or self-report measures. In a recent Danish follow-up of 151 anorectic patients (Brinch, Isager, & Tolstrup, 1988), 50 of 140 women had borne children during the follow-up interval (mean, 12.5 years), while none of the 11 males had fathered a child. The patients were older at age of first delivery than the national average by 2 years (26.1 years vs. 24.1 years), and the number of children per woman for the patients was 0.6, compared to the national average of 1.7 for women aged 32. Of the 50 women who had borne children, 36 were considered to have recovered when they bore their child, and overall the mothers had a better outcome than the nonmothers. In the offspring, perinatal complications were common, prematurity was twice the expected rate, and perinatal mortality was six times the expected rate. Unfortunately, the authors did not report on such details as whether the higher perinatal mortality was related to the mothers' clinical status. Apparently most of the mothers did well during the pregnancy and the postpartum period. In a study of five anorectic women who had conceived while still below optimal weight, Treasure and Russell (1988) found impaired fetal growth and small babies at birth, although they demonstrated "catch-up" growth in the neonatal period. Prenatal complications in this relatively small series were not remarkable.

In summary, it would appear that women who have recovered from anorexia nervosa also have a better psychosexual adjustment than those who have not recovered. The high prematurity and perinatal mortality of children born to anorectic women should clearly be studied further.

All the studies reported that most patients were employed full-time at follow-up, with figures ranging from 68% (Hall et al., 1984) to 78% (Hsu et al., 1979). Eighty-one percent of the males in the Burns and Crisp series were employed. Conversely, unemployment figures were low, ranging from 4% (Hall et al., 1984) to 11% (Burns & Crisp, 1984). Even emaciated patients were often fully or partially employed. Economic productivity is thus an area spared by the anorectic illness. Other areas of psychosocial adjustment, such as relationship with family, are difficult to assess objectively. The use of standardized measures and the inclusion of a control population are strongly recommended for future studies.

Prognostic Indicators

Five factors were found by at least three of the studies to indicate poor outcome: longer duration of illness, lower minimum weight, premorbid personality and social difficulties, disturbed relationship with family, and previous treatment (see Table 7.5). Theander (1970) found a later age of onset and vomiting to indicate poor outcome, but his outcome measures were somewhat different. A longer duration of illness, lower weight, and failed previous treatment are likely to be indices of chronicity, and in Patton's study (Patton, 1988a) lower weight and failed previous treatment also predicted fatal outcome. Poor premorbid social adjustment, perhaps a measure of personality strength and social adaptability, also predicts poor outcome in schizophrenia (Cutting, 1986). However, the precise significance of this finding for anorexia nervosa is still unclear, since all the studies were retrospective and none used standardized instruments to measure personality and social adjustment. How poor family interaction could lead to chronicity is unclear; perhaps it operates through "negative expressed emotion," a concept found useful in predicting relapse for both schizophrenia and depressive neurosis (Leff & Vaughn, 1980). In a study of parental expressed emotion in the families of 51 anorectics and bulimics, Szmukler and colleagues (1985) found parental critical comments to correlate with early dropout from treatment. However, the investigators did not report on the association between negative expressed emotion and outcome of illness.

Long-Term Outcome of Anorexia Nervosa and Treatment Effects

Russell (1970) originally suggested that a follow-up of at least 4 years was probably necessary for the anorectic illness to run its full course.

TABLE 7.5. Prognostic Indicators (Factors Associated with Poor Outcome)

	Burns & Crisp (1984)	Hall et al. (1984)	Hsu et al. (1979)	Morgan et al. (1983)	Morgan & Russell (1975)
Longer duration of illness	X		X	X	X
Lower minimum weight	X		X		X
Later age of onset	Possible		X		X
Vomiting		Possible	X		
Being married		X	X		
Personality/social difficulties	Possible		X	X	X
Disturbed relationship with family	X		X	X	X
Previous treatment	X		X		X

199

Two of the long-term (20 year) follow-up studies (Russell, personal communication, October 23, 1989; Theander, 1985), however, suggest otherwise. The longer the follow-up, the more the patients who have recovered, but also the more who have died. This is well illustrated by Theander's (1985) study of his original 94 patients (Theander, 1970). At 5 years after onset of illness, 18% had a poor outcome and 8% had died. At 33 years after onset, the figures were 6% and 18%, respectively. Thus those who remain ill at 5 years may run a significant risk of succumbing to the illness in the long run: Of the seven patients who were anorectic in 1966, four had died by 1980 and two of the remaining three were still severely anorectic. Of those who recovered, about one-third each did so by 3, 6, and 12 years after onset, respectively. Recovery after 12 years of continuous illness is therefore rare, although not impossible (see "Treating Chronic Patients," Chapter 6). The most common causes of death were starvation (12/17) and suicide (5/17). Two-thirds (11/17, or 12% of all 94 patients involved in the study) of the deaths in this study occurred within the first 7 years after onset of illness.

Russell (personal communication, October 23, 1989) restudied his 41 patients 20 years after their discharge from the Maudsley hospital and found a mortality rate of 15% (6/41, a seventh patient died of causes unrelated to anorexia nervosa), as compared to 5% at 4 to 10 years follow-up. However, the recent St. George's Hospital data (Crisp & Hsu, unpublished) do not indicate a significant increase in mortality over time: at 20-year follow-up the mortality rate was 4% (4/105), as compared to 2% (2/105) at 4 to 8 years follow-up. Furthermore, the cause of death (bronchial carcinoma) of one patient was not directly related to anorexia nervosa.

Because none of the studies mentioned above were designed as prospective treatment studies, no definitive conclusion can be drawn regarding the effect of treatment on outcome. Nevertheless, the low mortality rate (0% to 1%) in the three most recent intermediate-term outcome studies (Burns & Crisp, 1984; Hall, Slim, Hawker, & Salmond, 1984; Morgan, Purgold, & Welbourne, 1983) is striking, with the data seeming to support Crisp's contention (1981) that competent treatment may result in a decrease at least in early mortality. Furthermore, since the St. George's cohort (Crisp, Hsu, Harding, & Hartshorn, 1980; Hsu, Crisp, & Harding, 1979) was not different in terms of chronicity or severity of illness to the Maudsley (Morgan & Russell, 1975) or the

Swedish (Theander, 1970, 1985) cohort, their relatively low long-term mortality rate is particularly intriguing. It is tempting, although premature, to ascribe it to a treatment effect. It will be of great importance to determine if the mortality rate of the three other cohorts (Burns & Crisp, 1984; Hall et al., 1984; Morgan et al., 1983) increases with time. If it does not, then I think that the case that competent treatment does improve outcome will become stronger.

OUTCOME OF BULIMIA NERVOSA

To the best of my knowledge, there are 13 short-term (at least 12 months) outcome studies for bulimia nervosa (Abraham, Myra, Llewellyn-Jones, 1983; Fairburn, 1981; Fairburn et al., 1986; Hsu & Holder, 1986; Hsu & Sobkiewicz, in press-b; Huon & Brown, 1985; Johnson et al., 1986; Lacey, 1983; Mitchell et al., 1989; Russell et al., 1987; Swift et al., 1987; Wilson et al., 1986; Yager, Landsverk & Edelstein, 1987) (see Table 7.6). Except for the study by Yager and colleagues (1987), all were treatment and outcome studies. Patients in two studies (Russell et al., 1987; Swift et al., 1987) were treated initially as inpatients, followed by outpatient treatment. Russell and colleagues (1987) randomized their patients to individual supportive versus family therapy, while the patients in the series by Swift and colleagues (1987) received nonspecific inpatient treatment. Patients in the other ten studies were given outpatient, cognitive–behavioral treatment of varying intensity and duration. All the patients were normal-weight bulimics, the only exception being those in Russell and colleagues' (1987) study, all of whom suffered from a combination of bulimia nervosa and anorexia nervosa.

Direct comparison between studies of bulimic behavior at follow-up is difficult because different criteria were used to measure outcome. For instance, Russell and colleagues (1987) applied a strict criteria, rating even patients with occasional binges of less than once a week as having an intermediate outcome, whereas Hsu and Holder (1986) would have classified these patients as having made a good recovery. Fortunately, almost all the studies reported in detail on their outcome findings and clearly defined the outcome criteria; thus in most instances we can apply the *DSM-III-R* criterion of two episodes per week for the rating of outcome.

TABLE 7.6. Outcome of Bulimia Nervosa

Author	N/N Followed	Treatment[a]	Duration (months)	Method	Bulimia Nervosa[b] nondiagnosable (%)	Diagnosable (%)	Further body weight	Treatment
Abraham et al. (1983)	51/43	OP, I	14–72	Interview	65 (?)	35 (?)	Normal	ND
Fairburn (1981)	11/6	OP, I	12	ND[c]	83	17	Normal	None
Fairburn et al. (1986)	24/22	OP, I	12	Interview	100	—	Normal	None
Hsu & Holder (1986)	56/48	OP, I	12–35	Telephone	75	25	Normal	ND
Hsu & Sobkiewicz (in press-b)	45/35	OP, I	48–60	Mostly telephone	47	16 (16% symptomatic but nondiagnosable)	Normal 2% underweight	30%
Huon & Brown (1985)	45/40	OP, G	6–18	ND	90 (?)	5(?)	ND	ND
Johnson et al. (1986)	12/6	OP, I	12	ND	83	17	ND	ND
Lacey (1983)	30/28	OP, I, G	Up to 24	ND	100	—	Normal	11%
Mitchell et al. (1989)	100/91	OP, G	24–60	Telephone	66	25 (9% symptomatic but nondiagnosable)	Normal 1% underweight 7% overweight	ND
Russell et al. (1987)	23/23	IP, OP, I, F	12	Interview	At least 21	ND	Mostly normal	ND
Swift et al. (1987)	38/30	IP, OP (?)	24–60	Interview	50	50	Normal	100%
Wilson et al. (1986)	17/11	OP, G	12	Interview	73	27	Normal	36%
Yager et al. (1987)	?/392	ND	20	Postal questionnaire	43 (?)	57 (?)	ND	ND

[a]OP = outpatient, IP = inpatient, I = individual, G = group, F = family.
[b]Percentages are based on patients successfully traced for follow-up.
[c]ND = not described.

Based on these studies, the short-term outcome of bulimia nervosa is encouraging: At least two-thirds of the patients were no longer diagnosable as suffering from bulimia nervosa at 1-year follow-up according to the *DSM-III-R* frequency criterion. Body-weight change was minimal, and recovery from the illness was almost never associated with massive weight gain. Regression to restrictive anorexia nervosa was also rare, and control of the bingeing and purging was not associated with increased fasting. These findings were also true for the two intermediate-term outcome studies (Hsu & Sobkiewicz, in press-b; Mitchell et al., 1989).

However, there are some discrepancies in the studies' findings. The poorer outcome in the studies by Russell and colleagues (1987) and Yager and colleagues (1987) are perhaps explainable by patient-selection factors, the former group consisting of low-weight bulimics and the latter of nonclinic subjects. The stricter criteria of Russell and colleagues (1987), already mentioned, is clearly another factor that influenced their findings. Perhaps a third factor is treatment effect. If cognitive–behavioral techniques are indeed more effective than non-specific supportive treatment (see Chapter 6), the use of the latter may explain the relatively poor outcome in the studies of Yager and colleagues (1987) and Swift and colleagues (1987). It may also explain the better outcome in the several studies that used specific behavioral techniques (e.g., Fairburn et al., 1986). A fourth factor may have been variations in the length of follow-up duration; shorter follow-up might not have allowed the bulimic illness to run its full course.

Mental Status at Outcome

Studies that used standardized self-report measures found significant improvement in overall psychopathology; in particular, improvement in bulimic behavior (e.g., Johnson et al., 1986; Wilson et al., 1986) was accompanied by significant improvement in levels of depression and social anxiety. However, self-report of depression seemed to be common among those who were still bulimic (Hsu & Sobkiewicz, in press-b). Eating attitudes also improved significantly with recovery from the bulimic illness (Fairburn et al., 1986; Wilson et al., 1986). Using a standardized interview schedule (SADS-C), Swift and colleagues (1987) found none of the patients at follow-up to meet criteria for major depression or schizophrenia, nor did any novel psychiatric disorders emerge during the follow-up period. However, they found that in some patients suicide attempts, self-injurious behavior, shop-lifting, and alcohol abuse may have persisted despite improvement in bulimic behavior.

Mortality

None of the 13 studies reported any deaths at follow-up. In the study by Patton (1988a), three deaths occurred among the 96 normal-weight bulimics, two in traffic accidents and one following a severe weight loss. This represented a 940% increase over the expected mortality. While these figures need to be confirmed by other studies, they constitute a source of serious concern for those involved in the treat-ment of these patients.

Prognostic Indicators

Very few studies specifically addressed the issues of prognostic indica-tors for bulimia nervosa. Specifically, a previous history of anorexia nervosa was not predictive of outcome (Hsu & Holder, 1986; Lacey, 1983). This finding supports my view that it is unnecessary to include a history of anorexia nervosa as a diagnostic criterion. Hsu and Holder (1986) found longer duration of illness and positive family history of alcoholism and depression to predict poor outcome. While the former represents an index of chronicity, the latter could not be readily explained. When Mitchell and colleagues (1989) compared the best with the worst outcome group, they found a higher frequency of bingeing and vomiting at presentation to characterize the latter group. However, more severe depression at presentation was not asso-ciated with poor outcome. Clearly more data are needed.

THE NOSOLOGY OF THE EATING DISORDERS

Having reviewed the outcome studies of both anorexia nervosa and bulimia nervosa, I now return to the two overarching questions: Are the eating disorders simply variants of an affective illlness? Are they separate and distinct from each other?

Russell (1970) has suggested that the constancy of the association of the various clinical features and the fact that the illness runs
true-to-form are strong arguments for viewing anorexia nervosa as a
diagnostic entity. As already mentioned, none of the anorexia nervosa
outcome studies used a standardized instrument for the assessment of
mental state at outcome. Only Hall and colleagues (1984) used
DSM-III criteria to classify the diagnostic categories. They found that
dysthymic disorder was predominantly (15/17) associated with poor
or intermediate outcome and that major depression was uncommon.
The other investigators also found that depressive features most commonly occurred in those who were still anorectic. For instance, using
the Crown–Crisp Experiential Index (a self-report measure of psychiatric symptoms) at presentation and follow-up, Hsu and Crisp (1980)
found that recovery from the anorectic illness was associated with a
significant decrease in depression scores, while for those who were still
anorectic the scores remained the same. I have recently reanalyzed
the outcome data on a series of 50 anorectic patients that I had
reported earlier (Hsu, 1978). On retrospective analysis of the case
summaries of the 18 patients who reported depressive symptoms at
follow-up, I found that 6 could be assigned the following DSM-III
diagnoses: major depression (2), bipolar disorder (1), schizoaffective
disorder (1), obsessive–compulsive disorder (1), and social phobia (1).
Apart from the 1 patient with bipolar disorder, none of the other 5
patients had any significant anorectic or bulimic symptoms. Of the
remaining 12 patients with depressive symptoms not severe enough to
qualify for DSM-III major depression, 5 qualified for a diagnosis of
bulimia nervosa at normal weight, 3 for bulimic anorexia nervosa,
3 for restrictive anorexia nervosa; only 1 was free from any eating-
disorder symptoms. Even allowing for the limitations of a retrospective analysis, the evidence suggests that (1) minor depressive features
occur predominantly in those with a chronic eating disorder and
(2) for those who have recovered from anorexia nervosa, normal-
weight bulimia nervosa (not major depression) is the most common
diagnosis. The limited data available for bulimia nervosa also indicate
that depressive symptoms are more common for those who remain
bulimic.

Strober and Katz (1987), addressing the issue of nosological
relationship between affective and eating disorders, suggested that

depression may represent a final common pathway for many chronic psychiatric disorders not genetically related to one another, such as alcoholism, antisocial personality disorder, and schizophrenia. The evidence from the intermediate outcome studies certainly does not support the view that either anorexia nervosa or bulimia nervosa changes, in time, into major depression. Finally, the long-term course of anorexia nervosa in Theander's study (1985) does not at all resemble that of an affective illness (Keller, 1985).

We turn next to the association of bulimic and anorectic symptoms. At presentation or admission, bulimia (undefined) occurred in 38% (Hall et al., 1984) to 44% (Burns & Crisp, 1984; Hsu et al., 1979) of the patients in the five studies on anorexia nervosa, and vomiting occurred in 27% (Morgan & Russell, 1975) to 42% (Hsu et al., 1979). Since the frequency of such episodes was not described, it is unclear how many would also qualify for a *DSM-III-R* diagnosis of bulimia nervosa (i.e., more than two episodes per week). At follow-up Hsu and colleagues (1979), using a criterion of three or more episodes a week, found 19% to have bulimia and 21%, vomiting; thus at least 19% of the patients would qualify for *DSM-III-R* bulimia nervosa. Burns and Crisp (1984) found only 7% to have bulimia at follow-up and 10% to have vomiting, while Hall and colleagues (1984) reported that perhaps 38% of the patients had at least occasional bulimia and vomiting at follow-up. However, the frequency of these episodes was not specified.

Clearly, some patients lost their bulimia while others gained it from presentation to follow-up. Hall and colleagues (1984) reported that 6 lost it while 8 gained it. Hsu (1978), studying the first 50 of the 105 patients that he and colleagues later reported on in 1979 (Hsu, Crisp, & Harding, 1979), found 23 (46%) initially to have bulimia at presentation (frequency of symptoms unknown). At follow-up, 7 of the 23 bulimics (30%, including the 2 who had died) still had frequent (i.e., more than three times a week) bulimic and vomiting episodes, 8 (35%)had lost their bulimia, and the remaining 8 (35%) had binged and purged occasionally during the 6 months prior to follow-up. Thus the majority of bulimic anorectics continued to have an eating disorder at follow-up, with two-thirds (15/23) retaining their bulimia in varying degrees of severity. Only 3 (13%) had changed from bulimic to restrictive anorexia nervosa, and 5 (22%) had recovered, displaying neither anorexia nor bulimia nervosa. In contrast, of the 27 restrictive anorectics at follow-up, 7 (26%) had developed bulimia of varying severity and in the process also gained weight (i.e., developed bulimia nervosa at normal weight), 3 (11%) remained restrictive anorectics, and 17 (63%) had recovered, displaying no diagnosable eating disorder. To summarize: (1) With time, twice as many restrictive anorectics developed bulimia as bulimic anorectics developed restrictive anorexia; (2) most bulimic anorectics retained their bulimia; (3) restrictive anorectics who developed bulimia tended to gain weight (i.e., develop normal-weight bulimia nervosa), while bulimic anorectics tended to remain bulimic anorectics; (4) bulimia nervosa, normal-weight or otherwise, was the most common diagnosis after anorexia nervosa at follow-up; and (5) restrictive anorectics had a much better prognosis in terms of nutritional outcome.

The *DSM-III-R* provides no weight criteria for bulimia nervosa, nor did Russell (1979), who originally proposed the term. A patient at 85% of average weight (having lost, say, 20% of original weight) who binges and vomits three times a week will, according to the *DSM-III-R*, be given either a diagnosis of both anorexia nervosa and bulimia nervosa or a diagnosis of bulimia nervosa alone. Extending the criteria for bulimia nervosa to include that of low body weight is unsatisfactory for two reasons:

1. There is good evidence from the outcome studies reviewed above that the anorexia nervosa vomiting subgroup runs true-to-form, and available evidence suggests that normal weight bulimia nervosa does the same.

2. The treatment principles of the two disorders are different; weight gain is usually mandatory for the bulimic anorectic, if only to prevent death, but weight gain for the normal-weight bulimic is not necessary. Since a diagnosis usually carries some treatment implications, to give the same diagnosis to two disorders that require different treatment breeds ambiguity.

Therefore I suggest that anorexia nervosa be subdivided into the restricting (or abstaining) subgroup and vomiting (or bulimic) subgroup and that restriction of bulimia nervosa to normal-weight individuals be retained.

CONCLUSION

Recent outcome studies have found the intermediate-term outcome of anorexia nervosa to be relatively encouraging: From one-half to two-thirds of the patients have regained normal weight, and the overall mortality rate is below 5%. However, a chaotic eating pattern and morbid preoccupation with weight and food still affect almost two-thirds of the patients, even those who have regained normal weight. A substantial minority of the patients would qualify for a diagnosis of bulimia nervosa. In time, some of the chronic patients may succumb to the effects of starvation and some may commit suicide, so that the crude mortality rate at 20-year follow-up may be as high as 15% to 20%. Overall adjustment and mental status parallel weight and nutritional recovery. The evidence that patients recover from anorexia nervosa only to develop a major depression is not strong.

The outcome of bulimia nervosa has not been extensively studied. Overall it would appear that the short-term outcome of the illness is encouraging, with at least 50% of the patients no longer qualifying for a diagnosis of bulimia nervosa at 1- to 2-year follow-up. Long-term outcome is unknown. Mortality may be increased, but so far firm documentation is lacking. Again, improvement in overall adjustment occurs largely in tandem with the improvement in eating behavior.

These findings tell us that we should not confuse short-term improvement with long-term cure. They also tell us that there is a great need for vigorous treatment and outcome studies. For anorexia nervosa, there is some indication that active treatment may have prevented some early or even late deaths. The persistence of the eating disturbance in many patients, even those who are weight-recovered, should make us search for more specific treatments. The high long-term mortality rate indicates the importance of relapse prevention and the need to follow these patients carefully. For bulimia nervosa, the effectiveness over the short term of both cognitive–behavioral therapy and antidepressants is gratifying, but the need for long-term treatment and outcome studies should not be overlooked.

Epilogue

I have traced the historical development of the concept of the eating disorders, stated my position on the identities of anorexia nervosa and bulimia nervosa, described their clinical features, and presented my understanding of their epidemiology, etiology, diagnosis, treatment, and outcome. Here I briefly discuss primary prevention of the eating disorders and what I consider to be the direction of future research.

Primary prevention of the eating disorders (i.e., the prevention of their actual onset) is theoretically possible given the fact that we have identified the at-risk population and some of the risk factors involved in the pathogenesis of the disorders. For instance, if we could prevent a vulnerable individual from embarking on a rigorous and prolonged diet through nutritional counseling, then we might be able to prevent the onset of an eating disorder. Or we might attempt to decrease the pressure on women to be thin by changing the public's opinion of the ideal female. But how are we to accomplish this? Health professionals have rarely been very effective in changing public opinion, and societal preferences, particularly adolescent ones, do not usually change purely for health reasons. We cannot assume that educating the public on the eating disorders will necessarily result in primary prevention: A few of my patients actually claimed that they learned to vomit after watching educational programs on bulimia.

Will knowledge about what constitutes a healthy diet prevent a teenager from going on an unhealthy one to lose weight? Unfortunately there has been almost no research on the primary prevention of the eating disorders. Vandereycken and Meermann (1984) are pessimistic about the effectiveness of primary preventive measures, preferring instead to concentrate on secondary ones; that is, the early detection and treatment of cases. Crisp (1988) and Frankenburg, Garfinkel, and Garner (1982) are more optimistic, but they have not come forth with specific suggestions. I believe that the primary prevention of eating disorders should be carefully studied, beginning with identification of the risk factors through properly designed prospective studies, such as the one conducted by Patton (1988b). Nevertheless, I also believe that the many factors that enable the development of eating disorders are ultimately rooted in societal values, which are more "spiritual" (for want of a better word) in nature and thus unlikely to change as a result of empirical investigations. If so, then prevention may be a task that will require much more than simply an increase in scientific knowledge.

What, then, of the future? In exercising fantasy, I am reminded that in the not-so-distant past the steam locomotive was predicted to be the dominant mode of travel for twentieth-century man or that a cure of cancer was thought to be just around the corner. Nevertheless, some fantasies may generate healthy debate and stimulate fruitful research. Major breakthroughs are rare, and we can expect progress in our understanding of the eating disorders to be slow. Some research topics can be readily identified: the relationship between dieting behavior and weight change; outcome studies on diagnosable and subclinical cases that will allow us to better classify the eating disorders; prospective studies on high-risk populations that will clarify the risk factors involved in the pathogenesis of the disorders; and controlled treatment trials for both anorexia and bulimia nervosa that will yield more effective management strategies. However, progress in certain areas may be slow until advances are made on other fronts. For instance, a better understanding of the transmission of the eating disorders may not be possible until greater progress is made in the identification of genetic markers for psychiatric disorders, and efforts to maintain weight and control eating may not be very successful until we discover the central mechanisms involved in their regulation. In this regard, I predict that our understanding of the eating disorders will be more enhanced by advances in biomedical research than in psychosocial research. Finally, current research in related fields may point to new areas for our own research: studies in differential body fat distribution between the sexes (i.e., abdominal vs. gluteal-femoral) (e.g., Fried & Kral, 1987), studies in lipoprotein lipase activity (e.g., Hill, Thacker, Newby, Nickel, & Digirolamo, 1987), and studies on the effect of alternative fasting and overeating on food efficiency (ie.., ratio of weight gain to amount of energy ingested) (e.g., Reed, Contreras, Maggio, Greenwood, & Rodin, 1988) may have direct relevance to, for instance, why eating-disorder patients are particularly concerned about fat accumulation in the buttocks and upper thighs once they have gained some weight. I am therefore optimistic that a greater understanding of the pathogenesis, treatment, and outcome of the eating disorders will occur in the near future. I am less optimistic that this will result in a decrease in the overall magnitude of the problem of the eating disorders, since, as already mentioned, many of the issues involved in the development of an eating disorder are not readily changeable by better empirical research.

References

Numbers in parentheses following references refer to text pages on which they are cited (first citation in chapter).

Abraham, S., Bendit, N., Mason, C., Mitchell, H., O'Connor, N., Ward, J., Young, S., & Llewellyn-Jones, D. (1985). The psychosexual histories of young women with bulimia. *Australian and New Zealand Journal of Psychiatry, 19*, 72–76. (29)

Abraham, S., & Beumont, P. J. V. (1982a). How patients describe bulimia or binge eating. *Psychological Medicine, 12*, 625–635. (20)

Abraham, S., & Beumont, P. J. V. (1982b). Varieties of psychosexual experience in patients with anorexia nervosa. *International Journal of Eating Disorders, 1*, 10–19. (29)

Abraham, S., Myra, M., & Llewellyn-Jones, D. (1983). A study of outcome. *International Journal of Eating Disorders, 2*, 175–180. (201)

Agras, W. S., Barlow, D. H., Chapin, N. H., Abel, G., & Leitenberg, H. (1974). Behavior modification of anorexia nervosa. *Archives of General Psychiatry, 30*, 279–286. (137)

Agras, W. S., Dorian, B., Kirkley, B. G., Arnow, B., & Bachman, J. (1987). Imipramine in the treatment of bulimia: A double-blind controlled study. *International Journal of Eating Disorders, 6*, 29–38. (176)

Altshuter, K. Z., & Weiner, M. F. (1985). Anorexia nervosa and depression: A dissenting view. *American Journal of Psychiatry, 142*, 328–332. (9)

American Psychiatric Association. (1980). *Diagnostic and statistical manual of mental disorders* (3rd ed.). Washington, DC: Author. (4, 114)

American Psychiatric Association. (1987). *Diagnostic and statistical manual of mental disorders* (3rd ed., rev.). Washington, DC: Author. (4, 31, 114)

Andersen, A. E. (1985). *Practical comprehensive treatment of anorexia nervosa and bulimia.* Baltimore: Johns Hopkins University Press. (56, 135)

Andersen, A. E. (1987). Uses and potential misuses of antianxiety agents in the treatment of anorexia nervosa and bulimia nervosa. In P. E. Garfinkel &

D. M. Garner (Eds.), *The role of drug treatments for eating disorders* (pp. 59–89). New York: Brunner/Mazel. (151)

Andersen, A. E. (1988). Anorexia nervosa: Who are you? Where are you? *Mayo Clinic Procedures, 63,* 511–512. (64)

Askevold, F., & Heiberg, A. (1979). Anorexia nervosa: Two cases in discordant MZ twins. *Psychotherapy and Psychosomatics, 32,* 223–228. (89)

Bachman, G. A., & Kemmann, E. (1982). Prevalence of oligomenorrhea and amenorrhea in a college population. *American Journal of Obstetrics and Gynecology, 144,* 98–102. (25)

Baird, L. M., Silverstone, J. T., & Grimshaw, J. J. (1974). The prevalence of obesity in a London borough. *The Practitioner, 212,* 706–714. (79)

Barry, V. C., & Klawans, H. L. (1976). On the role of dopamine in the pathophysiology of anorexia nervosa. *Journal of Neural Transmission, 38,* 107–122. (54)

Beck, A. T. (1976). *Cognitive therapy and the emotional disorders.* New York: International Universities Press. (145)

Beck, A. T., Ward, C. H., Mendelson, M., Mock, J. E., & Erbaugh, J. K. (1961). An inventory for measuring depression. *Archives of General Psychiatry, 4,* 561–571. (110)

Beck, J. C., & Brochner-Mortensen, K. (1954). Observations on the prognosis in anorexia nervosa. *Acta Medica Scandinavica, 149,* 409–430. (23, 186)

Bell, R. M. (1985). *Holy anorexia.* Chicago: University of Chicago Press. (102)

Benjamin, L. (1974). Structural analysis of social behavior. *Psychological Review, 81,* 392–425. (39)

Bentovim, D. I., Marilov, V., & Crisp, A. H. (1979). Personality and mental state (p.s.e.) with anorexia nervosa. *Journal of Psychosomatic Research, 23,* 321–325. (9)

Bentovim, D. I., Whitehead, J., & Crisp, A. H. (1979). A controlled study of the perception of body width in anorexia nervosa. *Journal of Psychosomatic Research, 23,* 267–272. (22)

Beumont, P. J. V., Abraham, S. F., & Simson, K. G. (1981). The psychosexual histories of adolescent girls and young women with anorexia nervosa. *Psychological Medicine, 11,* 477–484. (24, 153)

Beumont, P. J. V., Abraham, S. F., & Turtle, J. (1980). Paradoxical response to LHRH during weight gain in patients with anorexia nervosa. *Journal of Clinical Endocrinology and Metabolism, 51,* 1283–1285. (49)

Beumont, P. J. V., George, G. C. W., & Smart, D. E. (1976). Dieters and vomiters and purgers in anorexia nervosa. *Psychological Medicine, 6,* 617–622. (3, 28)

Beutler, L. E., Crago, M., & Arizmendi, T. G. (1986). Research on therapist variables in psychotherapy. In S. L. Garfield & A. E. Bergin (Eds.), *Handbook of psychotherapy and behavior change* (pp. 257–310). New York: Wiley. (126)

Bhanji, S., & Thompson, J. (1974). Operant conditioning in the treatment of anorexia nervosa: A review and retrospective study of 11 cases. *British Journal of Psychiatry, 124,* 166–172. (140)

Biederman, J., Herzog, D. B., Rivinus, T. M., Ferber, R., Harper, G., Orsulak, P., Harmatz, J., & Schildkraut, J. (1984). Urinary MHPG in anorexia nervosa patients with and without a major depression disorder. *Journal of Psychiatric Research, 18,* 149-160. (54)

Biederman, J., Rivinus, T., Kemper, K., Hamilton, D., MacFadyen, J., & Harmatz, J. (1985). Depressive disorder in relatives of anorexia nervosa patients with and without a current episode of nonbipolar major depression. *American Journal of Psychiatry, 142,* 1495-1497. (34)

Blinder, B. J., Freeman, D. M. A., & Stunkard, A. J. (1970). Behavior therapy of anorexia nervosa: Effectiveness of activity as a reinforcer of weight gain. *American Journal of Psychiatry, 126,* 1093-1098. (130)

Bliss, E., & Branch, C. H. H. (Eds.). (1960). *Anorexia nervosa: Its history, psychology, and biology.* New York: Hoeber. (2, 187)

Bloom, R. E. (1983). The endorphins: A growing family of pharmacologically pertinent peptides. *Annual Review of Pharmacology and Toxicology, 23,* 151-170. (54)

Blos, P. (1970). *The young adolescent: Clinical studies.* London: Collier-MacMillan. (81)

Blouin, A. G., Blouin, J. H., Perez, E. L., Bushnik, T., Zuro, C., & Mulder, E. (1988). Treatment of bulimia with fenfluramine and desipramine. *Journal of Clinical Psychopharmacology, 8,* 261-269. (180)

Blumenthal, J. A., O'Toole, L. C., & Chang, J. L. (1984). Is running an analogue of anorexia nervosa? An empirical study of obligatory running and anorexia nervosa. *Journal of the American Medical Association, 252,* 520-523. (72)

Boskind-Lodahl, M. (1976). Cinderella's step-sister: A feminist perspective on anorexia nervosa and bulimia. *Signs: Journal of Women in Culture and Society, 2,* 342-356. (126)

Boskind-Lodahl, M., & White, W. C. (1978). The definition and treatment of bulimarexia in college women: A pilot study. *Journal of American College Health Association, 27,* 84-97. (4, 98)

Boyar, R. M., Katz, J., Finkelstein, J. W., Kapen, S., Weiner, H., Weitzman, E. D., & Hellman, L. (1974). Anorexia nervosa. Immaturity of the 24 hour luteinizing hormone secretory pattern. *New England Journal of Medicine, 291,* 861-865. (96)

Braddon, F. E. M., Rodgers, B., Wadsworth, M. E. J., & Davies, J. M. C. (1986). Onset of obesity in a 36 year birth cohort study. *British Medical Journal, 293,* 299-303. (79)

Branch, C. H. H., & Eurman, J. J. (1980). Social attitudes toward patients with anorexia nervosa. *American Journal of Psychiatry, 137,* 631-632. (80)

Brill, A. A. (1939). In discussion following: Pardoe, I. "Cachexia nervosa: A psychoneurotic simmonds syndrome." *Archives of Neurological Psychiatry, 41,* 842. (8)

Brinch, M., Isager, T., & Tolstrup, K. (1988). Anorexia nervosa and motherhood: Reproductional pattern and mothering behavior of 50 women. *Acta Psychiatrica Scandinavica, 77,* 90-104. (197)

Brooks-Gunn, J., & Matthews, W. S. (1979). *He and she: How children develop their sex role identity.* Englewood Cliffs, NJ: Prentice Hall. (84)

Brown, W. L. (1931). Anorexia nervosa. In W. L. Brown (Ed.), *Anorexia nervosa* (pp. 11-17). London: C. W. Daniels. (94)

Bruch, H. (1962). Perceptual and conceptual disturbances in anorexia nervosa. *Psychosomatic Medicine, 24,* 187-194. (12, 131, 144)

Bruch, H. (1964). Psychological aspects of overeating and obesity. *Psychosomatics, 5,* 269-274. (8)

Bruch, H. (1966). Anorexia nervosa and its differential diagnosis. *Journal of Nervous and Mental Disease, 141,* 555-566. (3)

Bruch, H. (1973). *Eating disorders: Obesity, anorexia nervosa, and the person within.* New York: Basic Books. (5, 23, 94, 131, 188)

Bruch, H. (1978). *The golden cage.* London: Open Books. (99, 129)

Bruch, H. (1982). Anorexia nervosa: Therapy and theory. *American Journal of Psychiatry, 132,* 1531-1538. (94, 132)

Bruch, H. (1985). Four decades of eating disorders. In D. M. Garner & P. E. Garfinkel (Eds.), *Handbook of psychotherapy for anorexia nervosa and bulimia* (pp. 7-18). New York: Guilford Press. (7, 87, 144)

Buhrich, N. (1981). Frequency of presentation of anorexia in Malaysia. *Australian and New Zealand Journal of Psychiatry, 15,* 153-155. (71)

Burns, T., & Crisp, A. H. (1984). Outcome of anorexia nervosa in males. *British Journal of Psychiatry, 145,* 319-325. (56, 189)

Bush, D. E., Simmons, R., Hutchinson, B., & Blyth, D. (1977-1978). Adolescent perceptions of sex roles in 1968 and 1975. *Public Opinion Quarterly, 41,* 459-474. (82)

Button, E. J., & Whitehouse, A. (1981). Subclinical anorexia nervosa. *Psychological Medicine, 11,* 509-516. (5, 65)

Cabellero, C. M., Giles, P., & Sharer, P. (1975). Sex role traditionalism and fear of success. *Sex Roles, 1,* 319-326. (86)

Calden, G., Lundy, R. M., & Schlater, R. J. (1959). Sex differences in body concepts. *Journal of Consulting Psychology, 23,* 378. (79)

Cantwell, D. P., & Baker, L. (1989). Anxiety disorders in adolescents. In L. K. G. Hsu & M. Hersen (Eds.), *Recent advances in adolescent psychiatry.* New York: Wiley. (104, 153)

Cantwell, D. P., Sturzenberger, S., Burroughs, J., Salkin, B., & Green, J. K. (1977). Anorexia nervosa: An affective disorder? *Archives of General Psychiatry, 34,* 1087-1093. (9, 94, 187)

Carlson, R. (1963). Identification and personality structure in preadolescents. *Journal of Abnormal Psychology, 67,* 566-573. (85)

Casper, R. C. (1982). Treatment principles in anorexia nervosa. *Adolescent Psychiatry, 10,* 431-454. (128)

Casper, R. C. (1987). Psychotherapy in anorexia nervosa. In P. J. V. Beumont, G. D. Burrows, & R. C. Casper (Eds.), *Handbook of eating disorders: Part 1. Anorexia and bulimia nervosa* (pp. 255-269). amsterdam: Elsevier. (132)

Casper, R. C., Eckert, E. D., Halmi, K. A., Goldberg, S. C., & Davis, J. M. (1980). Bulimia. *Archives of General Psychiatry, 37,* 1030-1035. (3)

Cattell, R. B., & Cattell, M. B. (1969). *Handbook for the high school personality questionnaire.* Champaign, IL: Institute for Personality and Ability Testing. (28)

Cavior, N., & Dokecki, P. (1973). Physical attractiveness, perceived attitude similarity, and academic achievement as contributors to interpersonal attraction among adolescents. *Developmental Psychology, 9,* 44–54. (80)

Cavior, N., & Lombardi, D. A. (1973). Developmental aspects of judgment of physical attractiveness in children. *Developmental Psychology, 8,* 67–71. (80)

Cecchin, G. (1987). Hypothesizing, circularity, and neutrality revisited: An invitation to curiosity. *Family Process, 26,* 405–413. (149)

Chang, K. S., Lee, M. M., & Low, W. D. (1963). Height and weight of Southern Chinese children in Hong Kong. *American Journal of Physiological Anthropology, 21,* 497–509. (78)

Chester, B. E. (1989). *Cognitive distortions in bulimia nervosa.* Unpublished manuscript. (168)

Christensen, U., Sonne-Holm, S., & Sorensen, T. I. A. (1981). Constant median body mass index of Danish young men, 1943–1977. *Human Biology, 53,* 403–410. (78)

Clarke, M. G., & Palmer, R. L. (1983). Eating attitudes and neurotic symptoms in university students. *British Journal of Psychiatry, 142,* 299–304. (68)

Cohen, D. J., Dibble, E., Grawe, J. M., & Pollin, W. (1973). Separating identical from fraternal twins. *Archives of General Psychiatry, 29,* 465–469. (90)

Cohen, D. J., Dibble, E., Grawe, J. M., & Pollin, W. (1975). Reliably separating identical from fraternal twins. *Archives of General Psychiatry, 32,* 1371–1375. (90)

Collins, M., Hodas, G. R., & Liebman, R. (1983). Interdisciplinary model for the inpatient treatment of adolescents with anorexia nervosa. *Journal of Adolescent Health Care, 4,* 3–8. (140)

Cooper, P. J., Charnock, D. J., & Taylor, M. J. (1987). The prevalence of bulimia nervosa: A replication study. *British Journal of Psychiatry, 151,* 684–686. (70)

Cooper, P. J., & Fairburn, C. G. (1983). Binge-eating and self-induced vomiting in the community: A preliminary study. *British Journal of Psychiatry, 142,* 139–144. (66, 160)

Cooper, P. J., & Fairburn, C. G. (1984). Cognitive behavior therapy for anorexia nervosa: Some preliminary findings. *Journal of Psychosomatic Research, 28,* 493–499. (157)

Cooper, P. J., & Fairburn, C. G. (1986). The depressive symptoms of bulimia nervosa. *British Journal of Psychiatry, 148,* 268–274. (9)

Copeland, J. (1981). What is a "case?" A case for what? In J. K. Wing, P. Bebbington, & L. N. Robins (Eds.), *What is a case? The problem of definition in psychiatric community surveys* (pp. 9–11). London: Grant McIntyre. (60)

Costello, A., Edelbrock, C., Dulcan, H., Kalas, R., & Klaric, S. (1980). *Diagnostic interview schedule for children (DISC).* Unpublished manuscript, Western Psychiatric Institute and Clinic, Pittsburgh, PA. (110)

Craigen, G., Kennedy, S., Garfinkel, P. E. & Jeejeebhoy, K. (1987). Drugs that facilitate gastric emptying. In P. E. Garfinkel & D. M. Garner (Eds.), *The role of drug treatments for eating disorders* (pp. 161–180). New York: Brunner/Mazel. (52)

Crighton-Miller, H. (1938). Prepsychotic anorexia. *Lancet, ii,* 1174. (9)

Cremerius, J. (1965). Zur prognose der anorexia nervosa. *Archiv fur Psychiatrie und Zeitschrift fur Neurologie, 207,* 378-393. (187)

Crisp, A. H. (1965). A treatment regime for anorexia nervosa. *British Journal of Psychiatry, 30,* 279-286. (27, 89, 151)

Crisp, A. H. (1967). Anorexia nervosa. *Hospital Medicine, 1,* 713-718. (3, 37, 84, 125)

Crisp, A. H. (1977). Diagnosis and outcome of anorexia nervosa. *Proceedings of the Royal Society of Medicine, 70,* 464-470. (37, 115, 189)

Crisp, A. H. (1980). *Anorexia nervosa: Let me be.* London: Plenum Press. (4, 28, 84, 125)

Crisp, A. H. (1981). Therapeutic outcome in anorexia nervosa. *Canadian Journal of Psychiatry, 26,* 232-235. (200)

Crisp, A. H. (1988). Some possible approaches to prevention of eating and body weight/shape disorders, with particular reference to anorexia nervosa. *International Journal of Eating Disorders, 7,* 1-17. (210)

Crisp, A. H., Burns, T., & Bhat, A. V. (1986). Primary anorexia nervosa in the male and female: A comparison of clinical features and prognosis. *British Journal of Medical Psychology, 59,* 123-132. (57)

Crisp, A. H., Ellis, J., & Lowry, C. (1967). Insulin response to a rapid intravenous injection of dextrose in patients with anorexia nervosa and obesity. *Postgraduate Medical Journal, 43,* 97-102. (10)

Crisp, A. H., Fenton, G. W., & Scotton, L. (1968). A controlled study of the EEG in anorexia nervosa. *British Journal of Psychiatry, 114,* 1149-1160. (41)

Crisp, A. H., Harding, B., & McGuinness, B. (1974). Psychoneurotic characteristics of parents: Relationship to prognosis. *Journal of Psychosomatic Research, 18,* 167-173. (37, 100)

Crisp, A. H., & Hsu, L. K. G. (1989). [Long-term outcome of anorexia nervosa— the St. George's Study]. Unpublished data. (200)

Crisp, A. H., Hsu, L. K. G., Chen, C. N., & Wheeler, M. (1982). Reproductive hormone profiles in male anorexia nervosa before, during and after restoration of body weight to normal: A study of twelve patients. *International Journal of Eating Disorders, 1,* 3-9. (57)

Crisp, A. H., Hsu, L. K. G., & Harding, B. (1980). The starving hoarder and voracious spender: Stealing in anorexia nervosa. *Journal of Psychosomatic Research, 24,* 225-231. (153)

Crisp, A. H., Hsu, L. K. G., Harding, B., & Hartshorn, J. (1980). Clinical features of anorexia nervosa. *Journal of Psychosomatic Research, 24,* 179-191. (7, 15, 70, 200)

Crisp, A. H., Norton, K. R. S., Jurczak, S., Bowyer, C., & Duncan, S. (1985). A treatment approach to anorexia nervosa—25 years on. *Journal of Psychiatric Research, 19,* 393-404. (125)

Crisp, A. H., Palmer, R. L., & Kalucy, R. S. (1976). How common is anorexia nervosa? A prevalence study. *British Journal of Psychiatry, 128,* 549-554. (165)

Crisp, A. H., & Stonehill, E. (1971). Relation between aspects of nutritional disturbance and menstrual activity in primary anorexia nervosa. *British Medical Journal, 3,* 149–151. (26)

Crisp, A. H., & Toms, D. A. (1972). Primary anorexia nervosa or weight phobia in the male. *British Medical Journal, i,* 334–338. (56, 91)

Cutting, J. (1986). Outcome of schizophrenia: Overview. In A. Kerr & P. Sanith (Eds.), *Contemporary issues in schizophrenia* (pp. 433–440). London: The Royal College of Psychiatrists. (198)

Dally, P. J. (1969). *Anorexia nervosa.* London: Heinemann. (8, 23, 115, 157)

Dally, P. J., & Sargant, W. (1960). A new treatment of anorexia nervosa. *British Medical Journal, 1,* 1770–1774. (130)

Darby, P. L., Garfinkel, P. E., Vale, J. M., Kirwan, P. J., & Brown G. M. (1981). Anorexia nervosa and turner syndrome: Cause or coincidence? *Psychological Medicine, 11,* 141–145. (40)

Dare, C. (1983). Family therapy for families containing an anorectic youngster. In *Understanding anorexia nervosa and bulimia* (pp. 28–36). (Report of the Fourth Ross Conference on Medical Research). Columbus, OH: Ross Laboratories. (156)

Derogatis, L. R., Lipman, R. S., & Covi, L. (1973). SCL-90: An outpatient psychiatric rating scale—A preliminary report. *Psychopharmacology Bulletin, 9,* 13–28. (82, 122)

Dixon, K. N., & Kiecolt-Glaser, J. (1984). Group therapy for bulimia. *Hillside Journal of Clinical Psychiatry, 6,* 156–170. (170)

Dornbusch, S. M., Carlsmith, J. M., Duncan, P. D., Gross, R. T., Martin, J. A., Ritter, P. L., & Siegel-Gorelick, B. (1984). Sexual maturation, social class, and the desire to be thin among adolescent females. *Developmental and Behavior Pediatrics, 5,* 308–314. (79)

Douvan, E., & Adelson, J. (1966). *The adolescent experience.* New York: Wiley. (86)

Driver, E. D., & Driver, A. E. (1983). Social class and height and weight in metropolitan madras. *Social Biology, 30,* 189–204. (78)

Druss, R. G., & Silverman, J. A. (1979). Body image and perfectionism of ballerinas. *General Hospital Psychiatry, 2,* 115–121. (71)

Dummer, G. M., Rosen, L. W., Heusner, W. W., Roberts, P. J., & Counsilman, J. E. (1987). Pathogenic weight control behavior of young, competitive swimmers. *Physician in Sports Medicine, 15,* 75–84. (72)

Eckert, E. D., Goldberg, S. C., Halmi, K. A., Casper, R. C., & Davis, J. M. (1979). Behavior therapy in anorexia nervosa. *British Journal of Psychiatry, 134,* 55–59. (142)

Eckert, E. D., Goldberg, S. C., Halmi, K. A., Casper, R. C., & Davis, J. M. (1982). Depression in anorexia nervosa. *Psychological Medication, 12,* 115–122. (9, 153)

Eisenberg, L. (1986). When is a case a case? In M. Rutter, C. E. Izard, & P. B. Read (Eds.), *Depression in young people* (pp. 469–478). New York: Guilford Press. (113)

Eisler, I., & Szmukler, G. I. (1985). Social class as a confounding variable in the eating attitudes test. *Journal of Psychiatric Research, 19,* 171–176. (65)

Elkin, T. C., Hersen, M., Eisler, R. M., & Williams, J. G. (1973). Modification of caloric intake in anorexia nervosa. *Psychological Report, 32,* 75–78. (141)

Ellis, A. (1962). *Reason and emotion in psychotherapy.* New York: Lyle Stuart. (167)

Enas, G., Pope, H., & Levine, L. (1989, May). *Fluoxetine in anorexia nervosa.* Paper (NR386) presented at the 142nd American Psychiatric Association Annual Meeting, San Francisco, CA. (178)

Endicott, J., & Spitzer, R. (1978). A diagnostic interview. *Archives of General Psychiatry, 35,* 837–844. (122)

Enns, M. P., Drewnowski, A., & Grinker, J. A. (1987). Body composition, body size estimation and attitudes towards eating in male college athletes. *Psychosomatic Medicine, 49,* 56–64. (72)

Erikson, E. H. (1955). The problem of ego identity. *Journal of Psychoanalytic Association, 4,* 56–121. (85)

Fairburn, C. G. (1981). A cognitive–behavioral approach to the management of bulimia. *Psychological Medicine, 11,* 707–711. (97, 161, 201)

Fairburn, C. G. (1982). Binge eating and its management. *British Journal of Psychiatry, 141,* 631–633. (163)

Fairburn, C. G. (1985). Cognitive–behavioral treatment for bulimia. In D. M. Garner & P. E. Garfinkel (Eds.), *Handbook of psychotherapy for anorexia nervosa and bulimia* (pp. 160–192). New York: Guilford Press. (160)

Fairburn, C. G., & Cooper, P. J. (1984). The clinical features of bulimia nervosa. *British Journal of Psychiatry, 144,* 238–246. (24)

Fairburn, C. G., Kirk, J., O'Connor, M., & Cooper, P. J. (1986). A comparison of two psychological treatments for bulimia nervosa. *Behavior Research and Therapy, 24,* 629–643. (166, 201)

Fallon, A. E., & Rosen, P. (1985). Sex differences in perceptions of desirable body shape. *Journal of Abnormal Psychology, 94,* 102–105. (79)

Faust, M. S. (1983). Alternative constructions of adolescent growth. In J. Brooks-Gunn & A. C. Petersen (Eds.), *Girls at puberty* (pp. 105–125). New York: Plenum Press. (85)

Fava, M., Copeland, P. M., Schweiger, U., & Herzog, D. B. (1989). Neurochemical abnormalities of anorexia nervosa and bulimia nervosa. *American Journal of Psychiatry, 146,* 963–971. (48)

Feighner, J. P., Robins, E., Guze, S. B., Woodruff, R., Winokur, G., & Munoz, R. (1972). Diagnostic criteria for use in psychiatric research. *Archives of General Psychiatry, 26,* 57–63. (3, 72, 114, 189)

Fenichel, O. (1945). *The psychoanalytic theory of neurosis.* London: Routledge & Kegan Paul. (9)

Finn, S. E., Hartman, M., Leon, G. R., & Larson, L. (1986). Eating disorders and sexual abuse: Lack of confirmation for a clinical hypothesis. *International Journal of Eating Disorders, 5,* 1051–1059. (23)

Foster, F. G., & Kupfer, D. J. (1975). Anorexia nervosa: Telemetric assessment of family interaction and hospital events. *Journal of Psychiatric Research, 12,* 19–35. (89)

Frankenburg, F., Garfinkel, P. E., & Garner, D. M. (1982). Anorexia nervosa: Issues in prevention. *Journal of Preventive Psychiatry, 1*, 469–483. (210)

Franklin, J. C., Schiele, B. C., Brozek, J., & Keys, A. (1948). Observations on human behavior in experimental semistarvation and rehabilitation. *Journal of Clinical Psychology, 4*, 28–45. (17)

Freeman, C., Sinclair, F., Turnbull, J., & Annadale, A. (1985). Psychotherapy for bulimia: A controlled study. *Journal of Psychiatric Research, 19*, 473–478. (171)

Fremouw, W. J., & Heyneman, N. E. (1984). A functional analysis of binge episodes. In R. C. Hawkins, W. J. Fremouw, & P. F. Clement (Eds.), *The binge–purge syndrome: Diagnosis, treatment, and research* (pp. 254–263). New York: Springer. (98)

Freud, A. (1958). Adolescence. *Psychoanalytic Study of Children, 13*, 255–278. (81)

Fried, S. K., & Kral, J. G. (1987). Sex differences in regional distribution of fat cell size and lipoprotein lipase activity in morbidly obese patients. *International Journal of Obesity, 11*, 129–149. (211)

Frisch, R. E., & McArthur, J. (1974). Menstrual cycles: Fatness as a determinant of minimum weight for height necessary for their maintenance or onset. *Science, 185*, 949–951. (96)

Frisch, R. E., Wyshak, G., & Vincent, L. (1980). Delayed menarche and amenorrhea in ballet dancers. *New England Journal of Medicine, 303*, 17–19. (96)

Furnham, A., & Alibhai, N. (1983). Cross-cultural differences in the perception of female body shapes. *Psychological Medicine, 13*, 829–837. (80)

Garb, J. L., Garb, J. R., & Stunkard, A. J. (1975). Social factors and obesity in Navaho Indian children. In A. Howard (Ed.), *Recent advances in obesity research* (pp. 37–39). London: Newman. (78)

Garfinkel, P. E., & Garner, D. M. (1982). *Anorexia nervosa: A multidimensional perspective.* New York: Basic Books. (40, 88, 131)

Garfinkel, P. E., Garner, D. M., Rose, J., Darby, P. L., Brandes, J. S., O'Hanlon, J., & Walsh, N. (1983). A comparison of characteristics in the families of patients with anorexia nervosa and normal controls. *Psychological Medicine, 13*, 821–828. (37)

Garfinkel, P. E., Kaplan, A. S., Garner, D. M., & Darby, P. L. (1983). The differentiation of vomiting/weight loss as a conversion disorder from anorexia nervosa. *American Journal of Psychiatry, 140*, 1019–1022. (120)

Garfinkel, P. E., Moldofsky, H., & Garner, D. M. (1977). The outcome of anorexia nervosa, significance of clinical features, body image, and behavior modification. In R. A. Vigersky (Ed.), *Anorexia nervosa* (pp. 315–329). New York: Raven Press. (188)

Garfinkel, P. E., Moldofsky, H., & Garner, D. M. (1980). The heterogeneity of anorexia nervosa. *Archives of General Psychiatry, 37*), 1036–1040. (3, 28)

Garn, S. M., & Clark, D. C. (1975). Nutrition, growth, development, and maturation: Findings from the Ten-State Nutrition Survey of 1968–1970. *Pediatrics, 56*, 306. (75)

Garn, S. M., & Clark, D. C. (1976). Trends in fatness and the origins of obesity. *Pediatrics, 57*, 443–456. (75)

Garner, D. M., & Bemis, K. M. (1982). A cognitive behavior approach to anorexia nervosa. *Cognitive Therapy and Research, 6,* 1-27. (97, 144)

Garner, D. M., & Bemis, K. M. (1985). Cognitive therapy for anorexia nervosa. In D. M. Garner & P. E. Garfinkel (Eds.). *Handbook of psychotherapy for anorexia nervosa and bulimia* (pp. 107-146). New York: Guilford Press. (97, 144)

Garner, D. M., Fairburn, C. G., & Davis, R. (1987). Cognitive-behavioral treatment of bulimia nervosa: A critical appraisal. *Behavior Modification, 11,* 398-431. (164)

Garner, D. M., & Garfinkel, P. E. (1979). The eating attitudes test: An index of the symptoms of anorexia nervosa. *Psychological Medicine, 9,* 273-279. (65, 80, 110)

Garner, D. M., & Garfinkel, P. E. (1980). Social-cultural factors in the development of anorexia nervosa. *Psychological Medicine, 10,* 647-656. (71)

Garner, D. M., Garfinkel, P. E., & Bemis, K. M. (1982). A multidimensional psychotherapy for anorexia nervosa. *International Journal of Eating Disorders, 1,* 3-46. (125)

Garner, D. M., Garfinkel, P. E., & O'Shaughnessy, M. (1985). The validity of the distinction between bulimics with and without anorexia nervosa. *American Journal of Psychiatry, 142,* 581-587. (7, 24)

Garner, D. M., Garfinkel, P. E., Rockert, W., & Olmsted, M. P. (1987). A prospective study of eating disturbances in the ballet. *Psychotherapy and Psychosomatics, 48,* 170-175. (72, 170)

Garner, D. M., Garfinkel, P. E., Schwartz, D., & Thompson, M. (1980). Cultural expectations of thinness in women. *Psychological Reports, 47,* 483-491. (80)

Garner, D. M., Olmsted, M. P., & Polivy, J. (1983). Development and validation of a multidimensional eating disorder inventory for anorexia nervosa and bulimia. *International Journal of Eating Disorders, 2,* 15-34. (76, 122)

Garner, D. M., Olmsted, M. P., Polivy, J., & Garfinkel, P. E. (1984). Comparison between weight-preoccupied women and anorexia nervosa. *Psychosomatic Medicine, 46,* 255-266. (5, 85)

Garner, D. M., Rockert, W., Olmsted, M. P., Johnson, C. L., & Coscina, D. V. (1985). Psychoeducational principles in the treatment of bulimia and anorexia nervosa. In D. M. Garner & P. E. Garfinkel (Eds.), *Handbook of psychotherapy for anorexia nervosa and bulimia* (pp. 513-572). New York: Guilford Press. (139)

Geracioti, T. D., & Liddle, R. A. (1988). Impaired cholecystokinin secretion in bulimia nervosa. *New England Journal of Medicine, 319,* 683-688. (56)

Gerner, R. H., Cohen, D. J., Fairbanks, L., Anderson, G. M., Young, J. G., Scheinin, M., Linnoila, M., Shaywitz, B. A., & Hare, T. A. (1984). CSF neurochemistry of women with anorexia nervosa and normal women. *American Journal of Psychiatry, 141,* 1441-1444. (54)

Gershon, E. S., Schreiber, J. L., Hamovit, J. R., Dibble, E. D., Kaye, W., Nurnberger, J. I., Andersen, A. E., & Ebert, M. (1984). Clinical findings in patients with anorexia nervosa and affective illness in their relatives. *American Journal of Psychiatry, 141,* 1419-1422. (33)

Gifford, S., Murawski, B. J., & Pilot, M. L. (1970). Anorexia nervosa in one of identical twins. *International Psychiatry Clinics, 7*, 139-228. (89)

Giles, T. R., Young, R. R., & Young, D. E. (1985). Case studies and clinical replication series: Behavioral treatment of severe bulimia. *Behavior Therapy, 16*, 393-405. (170)

Gillin, J. C., Duncan, W., Pettigrew, K. D., Frankel, B. L., & Snyder, F. (1979). Successful separation of depressed, normal, and insomniac subjects by EEG sleep data. *Archives of General Psychiatry, 36*, 85-90. (42)

Goldberg, S. C., Halmi, K. A., Eckert, E. D., Casper, R. C., & Davis, J. M. (1979). Cyproheptadine in anorexia nervosa. *British Journal of Psychiatry, 134*, 67-170. (152)

Goldblatt, P. B., Moore, M. E., & Stunkard, A. J. (1965). Social factors in obesity. *Journal of the American Medical Association, 192*, 1039-1044. (79)

Goodsitt, A. (1983). Self-regulatory disorders in eating disorders. *International Journal of Eating Disorders, 2*, 51-61. (96)

Goodsitt, A. (1985). Self-psychology and the treatment of anorexia nervosa. In D. M. Garner & P. E. Garfinkel (Eds.), *Handbook for psychotherapy for anorexia nervosa and bulimia* (pp. 55-82). New York: Guilford Press. (96, 135)

Gormally, J. (1984). The obese binge eater: Diagnosis, etiology, and clinical issues. In R. C. Hawkins, W. J. Fremouw, & P. F. Clement (Eds.), *The binge-purge syndrome: Diagnosis, treatment and research* (pp. 47-73). New York: Springer. (181)

Gormally, J., Black, S., Daston, S., & Rardin, D. (1982). Assessment of binge eating severity among obese persons. *Addictive Behaviors, 7*, 47-55. (181)

Graham, P., & Rutter, M. (1985). Adolescent disorders. In M. Rutter & L. Hersov (Eds.), *Child and adolescent psychiatry* (pp. 351-367). London: Blackwell. (82)

Gray, S. H. (1977). Social aspects of body image: Perception of normalcy of weight and affect of college undergraduates. *Perceptual and Motor Skills, 45*, 1035-1040. (83)

Green, R. S., & Rau, J. H. (1974). Treatment of compulsive eating disturbances with anticonvulsant medication. *American Journal of Psychiatry, 131*, 428-432. (179)

Grieve, W. P. (1946). Amenorrhoea during treatment. *British Medical Journal, ii*, 243-244. (25)

Griffin, M. E., Frazier, S. H., Robinson, D. B., & Johnson, A. M. (1957). The internist's role in the successful treatment of anorexia nervosa. *Proceedings of the Staff Meetings of the Mayo Clinic, 32*, 171-182. (138)

Grimshaw, L. (1959). Anorexia nervosa: A contribution to its psychogenesis. *British Journal of Medical Psychology, 32*, 44-49. (96)

Gross, H. A., Ebert, M. H., Faden, V. B., Goldberg, S. C., Lee, L. E., & Kaye, W. H. (1981). A double-blind controlled trial of lithium carbonate in primary anorexia nervosa. *Journal of Clinical Psychopharmacology, 1*, 376-381. (152)

Grounds, A. (1982). Transient psychosis in anorexia nervosa. *Psychological Medicine, 12,* 107–113. (153)

Gull, W. W. (1874). Anorexia nervosa (apepsia hysterica, anorexia hysterica). *Transactions of Clinical Society* (London), *7,* 22–28. (1, 56, 187)

Guyton, A. C. (1986). *Textbook of Medical Physiology* (5th ed., pp. 691–765). Philadelphia: W. B. Saunders. (52)

Hall, Alison (1985). Group psychotherapy for anorexia nervosa. In D. M. Garner & P. E. Garfinkel (Eds.), *Handbook of psychotherapy for anorexia nervosa and bulimia* (pp. 213–239). New York: Guilford Press. (150)

Hall, Alison, & Crisp, A. H. (1987). Brief psychotherapy in the treatment of anorexia nervosa outcome at one year. *British Journal of Psychiatry, 151,* 185–191. (139)

Hall, Anne (1978). Family structure and relationships of 50 female anorexia nervosa patients. *Australian and New Zealand Journal of Psychiatry, 12,* 263–268. (40)

Hall, Anne, Leibrich, J., Walkey, F. H., & Welch, G. (1986). Investigation of "weight pathology" of 58 mothers of anorexia nervosa patients and 204 mothers of schoolgirls. *Psychological Medicine, 16,* 71–76. (38)

Hall, Anne, Slim, E., Hawker, F., & Salmond, C. (1984). Anorexia nervosa: Long-term outcome in 50 female patients. *British Journal of Psychiatry, 145,* 407–413. (189)

Hall, G. S. (1891). The moral and religious training of children and adolescents. *Pedagogical Seminary, 1,* 196–210. (81)

Hallsten, E. A., Jr. (1965). Adolescent anorexia nervosa treated by desensitization. *Behavior Research and Therapy, 3,* 87–91. (142)

Hallstrom, T., & Noppa, H. (1981). Obesity in women in relation to mental illness, social factors and personality traits. *Journal of Psychosomatic Research, 25,* 75–82. (79)

Halmi, K. A. (1978). Anorexia nervosa: Recent investigations. *Annual Review of Medicine, 29,* 137–148. (41, 157)

Halmi, K. A. (1980). Anorexia nervosa. In H. I. Kaplan, A. M. Freedman, & B. J. Sadock (Eds.), *Comprehensive textbook of psychiatry* (Vol. 2, 3rd ed., pp. 1882–1890). Baltimore: Williams & Wilkins. (10)

Halmi, K. A. (1983). Treatment of anorexia nervosa. *Journal of Adolescent Health Care, 4,* 47–50. (124)

Halmi, K., & Brodland, G. (1973). Monozygotic twins concordant and discordant for anorexia nervosa. *Psychological Medicine, 3,* 521–524. (89)

Halmi, K., Brodland, G., & Loney, J. (1973). Progress in anorexia nervosa. *Annals of Internal Medicine, 78,* 907–909. (188)

Halmi, K. A., Casper, R., Eckert, E., Goldberg, S. C., & Davis, J. M. (1979). Unique features associated with age of onset of anorexia nervosa. *Psychiatry Research, 1,* 209–215. (22)

Halmi, K., Dekirmenjian, H., Davis, J. M., Casper, R., & Goldberg, S. (1978). Catecholamine metabolism in anorexia nervosa. *Archives of General Psychiatry, 35,* 458–460. (54)

Halmi, K. A., Eckert, E., LaDu, T. J., & Cohen, J. (1986). Anorexia nervosa: Treatment efficacy of cyproheptadine and amitriptyline. *Archives of General Psychiatry, 43,* 177-181. (152)

Halmi, K. A., Falk, J. R., & Schwartz, E. (1981). Binge-eating and vomiting: A survey of a college population. *Psychological Medicine, 11,* 697-706. (21, 66)

Halmi, K. A., Goldberg, S. C., Eckert, E., Casper, R., & Davis, J. M. (1977). Pretreatment evaluation in anorexia nervosa. In R. A. Vigersky (Ed.), *Anorexia nervosa* (pp. 43-54). New York: Raven Press. (40)

Halmi, K. A., Powers, P., & Cunningham, S. (1975). Treatment of anorexia nervosa with behavior modification. *Archives of General Psychiatry, 32,* 93-96. (140)

Halmi, K. A., Struss, A., & Goldberg, S. C. (1978). An investigation of weight in parents of anorexia nervosa patients. *Journal of Nervous and Mental Disorders, 166,* 358-359. (38, 79)

Hare, E. H., & Moran, P. A. P. (1979). Raised parental age in psychiatric patients: Evidence for the constitutional hypothesis. *British Journal of Psychiatry, 134,* 169-177. (40)

Hasan, M. K., & Tibbetts, R. W. (1977). Primary anorexia nervosa (weight phobia) in males. *Postgraduate Medical Journal, 53,* 146-151. (56)

Hawkins, R. C., II, & Clement, P. F. (1980). Development and construction validation of a self-report measure of binge eating tendencies. *Addictive Behaviors, 5,* 219-226. (163)

Healy, K., Conroy, R. M., & Walsh, N. (1985). Binge-eating and vomiting: A survey of a college population. *Psychological Medicine, 15,* 697-706. (66)

Heilbrun, A. B., Jr., Kleemeier, C., & Piccola, G. (1974). Developmental and situational correlates of achievement behavior in college females. *Journal of Personality, 42,* 420-436. (86)

Herman, C. P., & Polivy, J. (1975). Anxiety, restraint, and eating behavior. *Journal of Abnormal Psychology, 84,* 666-672. (97)

Herzog, D. B. (1984). Are anorexic and bulimic patients depressed? *American Journal of Psychiatry, 141,* 1594-1597. (9)

Herzog, D. B., & Copeland, P. M. (1988). Bulimia nervosa—Psyche and satiety. *New England Journal of Medicine, 319,* 716-718. (56)

Hill, J. O., & Holmbeck, G. N. (1987). Familial adaption to biological change during adolescence. In R. M. Lerner & T. T. Foch (Eds.), *Biological-psychosocial interactions in early adolescence* (pp. 207-223). New Jersey: Erlbaum. (84)

Hill, J. O., Thacker, S., Newby, D., Nickel, M., & Digirolamo, M. (1987). A comparison of constant feeding with bouts of fasting-refeeding at three levels of nutrition in the rat. *International Journal of Obesity, 11,* 251-262. (211)

Hoek, H. W., & Brook, F. G. (1985). Patterns of care of anorexia nervosa. *Journal of Psychiatric Research, 19,* 155-160. (62)

Hoffman, L. W. (1974). Fear of success in males and females: 1965-1972. *Journal of Consulting and Clinical Psychology, 42,* 353-358. (86)

Hogan, C. C. (1983). Psychodynamics. In C. P. Wilson (Ed.), *Fear of being fat* (pp. 115–128). New York: Jason Aronson. (131)

Holland, A. J., Hall, A., Murray, R., Russell, G. F. M., & Crisp, A. H. (1984). Anorexia nervosa: A study of 34 twin pairs and one set of triplets. *British Journal of Psychiatry, 145,* 414–418. (89)

Hollon, S., & Beck, A. T. (1986). Research on cognitive therapies. In S. L. Garfield & A. E. Bergin (Eds.), *Handbook of psychotherapy and behavior change* (pp. 443–482). New York: Wiley. (167)

Hooper, M. S. H., & Garner, D. M. (1986). Application of the eating disorders inventory to a sample of black, white, and mixed race schoolgirls in Zimbabwe. *International Journal of Eating Disorders, 5,* 161–168. (76)

Horner, M. (1968). *Sex differences in achievement motivation and performance in competive and noncompetitive situations.* Unpublished doctoral dissertation, University of Michigan, Ann Arbor. (86)

Hsu, L. K. G. (1978). *Anorexia nervosa: A prognostic study.* Unpublished dissertation for the degree of M.D., University of Hong Kong. (205)

Hsu, L. K. G. (1980). Outcome of anorexia nervosa: A review of the literature (1954–1978). *Archives of General Psychiatry, 37,* 1041–1046. (10, 153, 187)

Hsu, L. K. G. (1986). The treatment of anorexia nervosa. *American Journal of Psychiatry, 143,* 573–581. (117)

Hsu, L. K. G. (1987). Are the eating disorders becoming more common in blacks? *International Journal of Eating Disorders, 6,* 113–123. (70)

Hsu, L. K. G. (1988). The outcome of anorexia nervosa: A reappraisal. *Psychological Medicine, 18,* 807–812. (17, 142)

Hsu, L. K. G. (in press). Experiential aspects of bulimia nervosa: Implications for cognitive behavioral therapy. *Behavior Modification.* (20, 160)

Hsu, L. K. G., Chesler, B. E., & Santhouse, R. (in press). Bulimia nervosa in eleven sets of twins: A clinical report. *International Journal of Eating Disorders.* (90)

Hsu, L. K. G., Clement, L., Santhouse, R., Deep, D., & Ju, E. S. Y. (undated). *Treatment of bulimia nervosa with lithium carbonate: A controlled study.* Unpublished manuscript. (176, 180)

Hsu, L. K. G., & Crisp, A. H. (1980). The Crown–Crisp experiential index profile in anorexia nervosa. *British Journal of Psychiatry, 136,* 567–573. (9, 153, 205)

Hsu, L. K. G., Crisp, A. H., & Harding, B. (1979). Outcome of anorexia nervosa. *Lancet, i,* 62–65. (156, 188)

Hsu, L. K. G., & Holder, D. (1986). Bulimia nervosa: Treatment and short-term outcome. *Psychological Medicine, 16,* 65–70. (7, 16, 119, 160, 201)

Hsu, L. K. G., Holder, D., Hindmarsh, D., & Phelps, C. (1984). Bipolar illness preceded by anorexia nervosa in identical twins. *Journal of Clinical Psychiatry, 45,* 262–266. (88)

Hsu, L. K. G., & Lieberman, S. (1982). Paradoxical intention in the treatment of chronic anorexia nervosa. *American Journal of Psychiatry, 139,* 650–653. (158)

Hsu, L. K. G., Meltzer, E. S., & Crisp, A. H. (1981). Schizophrenia and anorexia nervosa. *Journal of Nervous and Mental Disorders, 169,* 273–276. (153)

Hsu, L. K. G., Milliones, J., Friedman, L., Holder, D., & Klepper, T. (1982,

October). *A survey of eating attitudes and behavior in adolescents.* Paper presented at the 25th Annual Meeting of the American Academy of Child Psychiatry, Washington, D.C. (75)

Hsu, L. K. G., & Sobkiewicz, T. A. (in press-a). Body image disturbance: Time to abandon the concept for eating disorders. *International Journal of Eating Disorders.* (12, 31)

Hsu, L. K. G. & Sobkiewicz, T. A. (in press-b). Bulimia nervosa: A 4 to 6 year follow-up study. *Psychological Medicine.* (94, 201)

Hsu, L. K. G., & Zimmer, B. (1988). Eating disorders in old age. *International Journal of Eating Disorders, 7,* 133–138. (22, 120)

Hudson, J. I., Pope, H. G., Jonas, J. M., Lipinski, J. F., & Kupfer, D. J. (1987). Electroencephalographic sleep in bulimia. In J. I. Hudson & H. G. Pope (Eds.), *The psychobiology of bulimia* (pp. 187–202). Washington, DC: American Psychiatric Press. (42)

Hudson, J., Pope, H., Jonas, J., & Yurgelun-Todd, D. (1983). Family history study of anorexia nervosa and bulimia. *British Journal of Psychiatry, 142,* 133–138. (33)

Hudson, J., Pope, H., Jonas, J., Yurgelun-Todd, D., & Frankenburg, F. R. (1987). A controlled family history study of bulimia. *Psychological Medicine, 17,* 883–890. (42)

Huenemann, R. L., Shapiro, L. R., Hampton, M. C., & Mitchell, B. W. (1966). A longitudinal study of gross body composition and body conformation and their association with food and activity in a teenage population. *American Journal of Clinical Nutrition, 18,* 325–338. (74)

Hughes, P. L., Wells, L. A., Cunningham, C. J., & Ilstrup, D. M. (1986). Treatment of bulimia with desipramine: A double-blind, placebo-controlled study. *Archives of General Psychiatry, 43,* 182–186. (176)

Humphrey, L. L. (1986a). Family relations in bulimic-anorexic and nondistressed families. *International Journal of Eating Disorders, 5,* 223–232. (39)

Humphrey, L. L. (1986b). Structural analysis of parent-child relationships in eating disorders. *Journal of Abnormal Psychology, 95,* 395–402. (39)

Humphrey, L. L. (1987). Comparison of bulimic-anorexic and nondistressed families using structural analysis of social behavior. *American Academy of Child and Adolescent Psychiatry, 26,* 248–255. (39, 95)

Huon, G. F., & Brown, L. B. (1985). Evaluating a group treatment for bulimia. *Journal of Psychiatric Research, 19,* 479–483. (161, 201)

Hurst, A. (1939). Discussion on anorexia nervosa. *Proceedings of the Royal Society of Medicine, 32,* 744–745. (187)

Huse, D. M., & Lucas, A. R. (1985). Treatment of anorexia nervosa: Dietary considerations. In R. T. Frankle, J. Dwyer, L. Moragne, & A. Owen (Eds.), *Dietary treatment and prevention of obesity* (pp. 201–210). London: Libbey. (134)

Isaacs, A. J. (1979). *Endocrinology in anorexia nervosa.* In P. Dally, J. Gomez, & A. J. Isaacs (Eds.), *Anorexia nervosa* (pp. 159–209). London: Heinemann. (10, 48)

Isner, J. M., Robert, W. C., Heymsfield, S. B., & Yager, J. (1985). Anorexia nervosa and sudden death. *Annals of Internal Medicine, 102,* 49–52. (157)

Jakobovits, C., Halstead, P., Kelley, L., Roe, D. A., & Young, C. M. (1977). Eating habits and nutrient intakes of college women over a thirty-year period. *Journal of the American Dietetic Association, 71,* 405–411. (75)

Jimerson, D. C., George, D. T., Kaye, W. H., Brewerton, T. D., & Goldstein, D. S. (1987). Norepinephrine regulation in bulimia. In J. I. Hudson & H. G. Pope (Eds.), *The psychobiology of bulimia* (pp. 147–156). Washington, DC: American Psychiatric Press. (56)

Johnson, C. (1985). Initial consultation for patients with bulimia and anorexia nervosa. In D. M. Garner & P. E. Garfinkel (Eds.), *Handbook of psychotherapy for anorexia nervosa and bulimia* (pp. 19–51). New York: Guilford Press. (110)

Johnson, C., & Connors, M. E. (Eds.). (1987). Demographic and clinical characteristics. *The etiology and treatment of bulimia nervosa. A biopsychosocial perspective* (pp. 31–60). New York: Basic Books. (29, 128)

Johnson, C., & Flach, A. (1985). Family characteristics of 105 patients with bulimia. *American Journal of Psychiatry, 142,* 1321–1324. (38)

Johnson, C. L., Lewis, C., Love, S., Lewis, L., & Studkey, M. (1983). *A descriptive survey of dieting and bulimic behavior in a female high school population* (pp. 14–18). (Report of the Fourth Ross Conference on Medical Research). Columbus, OH: Ross Laboratories. (66)

Johnson, C., Stuckey, M., Lewis, L., & Schwartz, D. (1982). Bulimia: A descriptive survey of 316 cases. *International Journal of Eating Disorders, 2,* 3–16. (24)

Johnson, W. G., Schlundt, D. G., & Jarrell, M. P. (1986). Exposure with response prevention, training in energy balance and problem solving therapy for bulimia nervosa. *International Journal of Eating Disorders, 5,* 35–45. (161, 201)

Johnson-Sabine, E., Wood, K., Patton, G., Mann, A., & Wakeling, A. (1988). Abnormal eating attitudes in London schoolgirls—A prospective epidemiological study: Factors associated with abnormal response on screening questionnaires. *Psychological Medicine, 18,* 615–622. (73)

Johnson-Sabine, E., Yonace, A., Farrington, A. J., Barrett, K. H., & Wakeling, A. (1983). Bulimia nervosa: A placebo-controlled double-blind therapeutic trial of mianserin. *British Journal of Clinical Pharmacology, 15*(Suppl.), 195–202. (175)

Jones, D. J., Fox, M. M., Babigan, H. M., & Hutton, H. E. (1980). Epidemiology of anorexia nervosa in Monroe County, New York: 1960–1976. *Psychosomatic Medicine, 42,* 551–558. (61)

Jones, M. C., & Mussen, P. H. (1958). Self-conceptions, motivations, and interpersonal attitudes of early- and late-maturing girls. *Child Development, 29,* 491–501. (84)

Jourard, S. E., & Secord, P. F. (1955). Body-cathexis and the ideal female figure. *Journal of Abnormal and Social Psychology, 50,* 243–246. (79)

Kalucy, R., Crisp, A. H., & Harding, B. (1977). A survey of 56 families with anorexia nervosa. *British Journal of Medical Psychology, 50,* 381–395. (23, 99)

Kandel, D. B., & Davies, M. (1982). Epidemiology of depressive mood in adolescents. *Archives of General Psychiatry, 39,* 1205–1212. (82)

Kaplan, A. S. (1987a). Thyroid function in bulimia. In J. I. Hudson & H. G. Pope (Eds.), *The psychobiology of bulimia* (pp. 15-28). Washington, DC: American Psychiatric Press. (55)

Kaplan, A. S. (1987b). Anticonvulsant treatment of eating disorders. In P. E. Garfinkel & D. M. Garner (Eds.), *The role of drug treatments for eating disorders* (pp. 96-123). New York: Brunner/Mazel. (42, 179)

Kaplan, S. L., Busner, J., & Pollack, S. (1988). Perceived weight, actual weight, and depressive symptoms in a general adolescent sample. *International Journal of Eating Disorders, 7,* 107-114. (83)

Kaplan, S. L., Nussbaum, M., Skomorowsky, P., Shenker, I. R., & Ramsey, P. (1980). Health habits and depression in adolescence. *Journal of Youth and Adolescence, 9,* 299-304. (83)

Katz, J. L., Boyar, R., Roffwarg, H., Hellman, L., & Weiner, H. (1978). Weight and circadian luteinizing hormone secretory pattern in anorexia nervosa. *Psychosomatic Medicine, 40,* 549-567. (26)

Katz, J. L., Kuperberg, A., Pollack, C. P., Walsh, B. T., Zumoff, B., & Weiner, H. (1984). Is there a relationship between eating disorder and affective disorder? New evidence from sleep recordings. *American Journal of Psychiatry, 141,* 753-759. (42)

Katzman, M. A., Wolchik, S. A., & Braver, S. L. (1984). The prevalence of frequent binge-eating and bulimia in a non-clinical college sample. *International Journal of Eating Disorders, 3,* 53-61. (66)

Kay, D. W. K., & Leigh, D. (1954). The natural history, treatment, and prognosis of anorexia nervosa based on a study of 38 patients. *Journal of Mental Science, 100,* 411-431. (3, 23)

Kaye, W. H. (1987). Opioid antagonist drugs in the treatment of anorexia nervosa. In P. E. Garfinkel & D. M. Garner (Eds.), *The role of drug treatments for eating disorders* (pp. 150-160). New York: Brunner/Mazel. (54)

Kaye, W. H., Ebert, M. H., Raleigh, M., & Lake, C. R. (1984). Abnormalities in CNS monoamine metabolism in anorexia nervosa. *Archives of General Psychiatry, 41,* 350-355. (54)

Kaye, W. H., Gwirtsman, H. E., George, D. T., Ebert, M. H., Jimerson, D. C., Tomai, T. P., Chrousos, G. P., & Gold, P. W. (1987). Elevated cerebrospinal fluid levels of immunoreactive corticotropin-releasing hormone in anorexia nervosa: Relation to state of nutrition, adrenal function, and intensity of depression. *Journal of Clinical Endocrinology and Metabolism, 54,* 203-208. (10)

Kaye, W. H., Gwirtsman, H. E., George, D. T., Jimerson, D. C., & Ebert, M. H. (1988). CSF 5-HIAA concentrations in anorexia nervosa: Reduced values in underweight subjects normalized after weight gain. *Biological Psychiatry, 23,* 102-105. (54)

Kaye, W. H., Gwirtsman, H. E., George, D. T., Weiss, S. R., & Jimerson, D. C. (1986). Relationship of mood alternatives to bingeing behavior in bulimia. *British Journal of Psychiatry, 149,* 470-485. (21)

Keller, M. B. (1985). Chronic and recurrent affective disorders: Incidence, course, and influencing factors. In D. Kemali & G. Racagni (Eds.), *Chronic treatments in neuropsychiatry* (pp. 111–120). New York: Raven. (10, 206)

Kendell, R. E. (1969). The continuum model of depressive illness. *Proceedings of the Royal Society of Medicine, 62,* 335–339. (11)

Kendell, R. E. (1975). *The role of diagnosis in psychiatry.* London: Blackwell. (11)

Kendell, R. E., Hall, D. J., Hailey, A., & Babigian, H. M. (1973). The epidemiology of anorexia nervosa. *Psychological Medicine, 3,* 200–203. (62)

Keys, A., Brozek, J., Henschel, A., Michelson, O., & Taylor, H. L. (1950). *The biology of human starvation: Vol I* (p. 828). Minneapolis, MN: University of Minnesota Press. (17, 161)

King, A. (1963). Primary and secondary anorexia nervosa. *British Journal of Psychiatry, 109,* 470–479. (38)

Kirkley, B. G., Schneider, J. A., Agras, W. S., & Bachman, J. A. (1985). Comparison of two group treatments for bulimia. *Journal of Consulting and Clinical Psychology, 53,* 43–48. (161)

Knuth, V. A., Hull, M. G. R., & Jacobs, H. S. (1977). Amenorrhea and loss of weight. *British Journal of Obstetrics and Gynaecology, 84,* 801–807. (26)

Kog, E. Vandereycken, W., & Vertommen, H. (1985). Towards a verification of the psychosomatic family model: A pilot study of ten families with an anorexia/bulimia nervosa patient. *International Journal of Eating Disorders, 4,* 525–538. (39)

Konopka, G. (1976). *Young girls: A portrait of adolescents.* Englewood Cliffs, NJ: Prentice-Hall. (86)

Kornhaber, A. K. (1970). The stuffing syndrome. *Psychosomatics, 11,* 580–584. (4)

Krieg, J. C., Pirke, K. M., Laver, C., & Backmund, H. (1988). Endocrine, metabolic, and cranial computed tomographic findings in anorexia nervosa. *Biological Psychiatry, 23,* 377–387. (42)

Kupfer, D., Foster, F., Reich, L., Thompson, K. S., & Weiss, B. (1976). EEG sleep changes as predictors in depression. *American Journal of Psychiatry, 138,* 429–434. (42)

Lacey, J. H. (1983). Bulimia nervosa, binge eating and psychogenetic vomiting: A controlled treatment study and long-term outcome. *British Medical Journal, 286,* 1609–1613. (7, 16, 119, 160, 201)

Lacey, J. H., & Crisp, A. H. (1980). Hunger, food intake and weight: The impact of clomipramine on a refeeding anorexia nervosa population. *Postgraduate Medical Journal, 56,* 79–85. (152)

Lasegue, E. C. (1873). On hysterical anorexia. *Medical Times Gazette, 2,* 265. (2, 99)

Lee, N. F., & Rush, P. A. J. (1986). Cognitive–behavioral group therapy for bulimia. *International Journal of Eating Disorders, 5,* 599–615. (170)

Lee, N. F., Rush, A. J., & Mitchell, J. E. (1985). Bulimia and depression. *Journal of Affective Disorders, 9,* 231–238. (9)

Leff, J. P., & Vaughn, C. E. (1980). The interaction of life events and relatives' expressed emotion in schizophrenia and depressive neurosis. *British Journal of Psychiatry, 136,* 146–153. (198)

Leibowitz, S. F., & Shor-Posner, G. (1986). Brain serotonin and eating behavior. *Appetite, 7* (Suppl.), 1–14. (52)

Leon, G. R., Lucas, A. R., Colligan, R. C., Ferndinande, R. J., & Kamp, J. (1985). Sexual, body image, and personality attitudes in anorexia nervosa. *Journal of Abnormal Child Psychology, 13,* 245–257. (29)

Lerner, R. M. (1969). The development of stereotype expectancies of body build–behavior relations. *Child Development, 40,* 137–141. (84)

Lerner, R. M., Iwawaki, S., Chihara, T., & Sovrell, G. T. (1980). Self-concept, self-esteem, and body attitudes among Japanese male and female adolescents. *Child Development, 51,* 847–855. (82)

Lerner, R. M., & Karabenick, S. A. (1974). Physical attractiveness, body attitudes and self-concept in late adolescents. *Journal of Youth and Adolescence, 3,* 307–316. (83)

Lesser, L. I., Asheden, B. J., Debriskey, M., & Eisenberg, L. (1960). Anorexia nervosa in children. *American Journal of Orthopsychiatry, 30,* 572–579. (11, 188)

Levenkron, S. (1983). *The best little girl in the world.* Chicago: Contemporary Books. (19, 145)

Levin, A. P., & Hyler, S. E. (1986). DSM-III personality diagnosis in bulimia. *Comprehensive Psychiatry, 27,* 47–53. (30, 97)

Levy, A. B., Dixon, K. N., & Malarkey, W. B. (1988). Pituitary response to TRH in bulimia. *Biological Psychiatry, 23,* 476–484. (55)

Levy, A. B., Dixon, K. N., & Schmidt, H. (1987). REM and delta sleep in anorexia nervosa and bulimia. *Psychiatry Research, 20,* 189–197. (42)

Lewin, K., Mattingly, D., & Millis, R. R. (1972). Anorexia nervosa associated with hypothalamic tumour. *British Medical Journal, ii,* 629–630. (40)

Loro, A. D., & Orleans, C. S. (1981). Binge eating in obesity: Preliminary findings and guidelines for behavioral analysis and treatment. *Addictive Behavior, 6,* 155–166. (163)

Lucas, A. R., Beard, C. M., O'Fallon, W. M., & Kurland, L. T. (1988). Anorexia nervosa in Rochester, Minnesota: A 45-year study. *Mayo Clinic Proceedings, 63,* 433–442. (61)

MacGregor, G. A., Markandu, N. D., Roulston, J. E., Jones, J. C., & de Wardener, H. E. (1979). Is "idiopathic" edema idiopathic? *Lancet, i,* 397–400. (157)

Maloney, M. J., & Farrell, M. K. (1980). Treatment of severe weight loss in anorexia nervosa with hyperalimentation and psychotherapy. *American Journal of Psychiatry, 137,* 310–314. (130)

Marrazzi, M. A., & Luby, E. D. (1986). An auto-addiction opioid model of chronic anorexia nervosa. *International Journal of Eating Disorders, 5,* 191–208. (151)

Masserman, J. H. (1941). Psychodynamics in anorexia nervosa and neurotic vomiting. *Psychoanalytical Quarterly, 10,* 211. (96)

McKay, M., Davis, M., & Fanning, P. (1981). Combating distorting thinking. In *Thoughts and feelings: The art of cognitive stress intervention* (pp. 17–45). Richmond, CA: New Harbinger Publications. (168)

Meichenbaum, D. (1977). *Cognitive–behavior modification.* New York: Plenum. (167)

Meyer, J. E. (1961). Das syndrom der anorexia nervosa. *Archiv fur Psychiatrie und Neurologie, 202,* 31–59. (3, 187)

Mills, I. H. (1976). Amitriptyline therapy in anorexia nervosa (letter). *Lancet, ii,* 687. (152)

Mintz, I. L. (1983). An analytic approach to hospital and nursing care. In C. P. Wilson (Ed.), *Fear of being fat: The treatment of anorexia and bulimia* (pp. 315–324). New York: Jason Aronson. (134)

Minuchin, S. (1974). *Families and family therapy.* Cambridge: Harvard University Press. (130)

Minuchin, S., Baker, L., Rosman, B. L., Liebman, R., Milman, L., & Todd, T. (1975). A conceptual model of psychosomatic illness in children. *Archives of General Psychiatry, 32,* 1031–1038. (99, 140)

Minuchin, S., & Fishman, H. C. (1981). *Family therapy techniques.* Massachusetts: Harvard University Press. (38, 99)

Minuchin, S., Rosman, B. L., & Baker, L. (1978). *Psychosomatic families.* Cambridge: Harvard University Press. (38, 109, 131, 187)

Mitchell, J. E., & Goff, G. (1984). A series of twelve adult male patients with bulimia. *Psychosomatics, 25,* 909–913. (57)

Mitchell, J. E., & Groat, E. (1984). A placebo-controlled, double-blind trial of amitriptyline in bulimia. *Journal of Clinical Psychopharmacology, 4,* 186–193. (175)

Mitchell, J. E., Hatsukami, D., Eckert, E. D., & Pyle, R. L. (1985). Characteristics of 275 patients with bulimia. *American Journal of Psychiatry, 142,* 482–485. (27, 160)

Mitchell, J. E., Hatsukami, D., Goff, G., Pyle, R. L., Eckert, E. D., & Davis, L. E. (1985). Intensive outpatient group treatment for bulimia. In D. M. Garner & P. E. Garfinkel (Eds.), *Handbook of psychotherapy for anorexia nervosa and bulimia* (pp. 240–253). New York: Guilford Press. (150)

Mitchell, J. E., Hatsukami, D., Pyle, R. L., & Eckert, E. D. (1986). What are atypical eating disorders? *Psychosomatics, 27,* 21–25. (29)

Mitchell, J. E., Hatsukami, D., Pyle, R. L., Eckert, E. D., & Soll, E. (1987). Late onset bulimia. *Comprehensive Psychiatry, 28,* 323–328. (22)

Mitchell, J. E., & Laine, D. C. (1985). Monitored binge-eating behavior in patients of normal weight with bulimia. *International Journal of Eating Disorders, 4,* 177–183. (20)

Mitchell, J. E., Morley, J. E., Levine, A. S., & Hatsukami, D. (1987). High-dose naltrexone therapy and dietary counseling for obesity. *Biological Psychiatry, 22,* 35–42. (56)

Mitchell, J. E., Pyle, R. L., Eckert, E. D., Hatsukami, D., & Lentz, R. (1983). Electrolyte and other physiological abnormalities in patients with bulimia. *Psychological Medicine, 13,* 273–278. (41)

Mitchell, J. E., Pyle, R. L., Hatsukami, D., Goff, G., Glotter, D., & Harper, J. (1989). A 2 to 5 year follow-up study of patients treated for bulimia. *International Journal of Eating Disorders, 8,* 157–165. (201)

Moos, R., & Moos, B. S. (1980). *Family environment scale manual*. Palo Alto: Consulting Psychologists Press. (38)

Morgan, G., & Sylvester, D. (1977). Anorexia nervosa. In O. W. Hill (Ed.), *Modern trends in psychological medicine* (Vol. 3, pp. 382–403). London: Butterworths. (67)

Morgan, H. G., & Russell, G. F. M. (1975). Value of family background and clinical features as predictors of long-term outcome in anorexia nervosa: Four year follow-up study of 41 patients. *Psychological Medicine, 5*, 355–371. (23, 134, 188)

Morgan, H. G., Purgold, J., & Welbourne, J. (1983). Management and outcome in anorexia nervosa: A standardized prognosis study. *British Journal of Psychiatry, 143*, 282–287. (131, 189)

Morley, J. E., & Blundell, J. E. (1988). The neurobiological basis of eating disorders: Some formulations. *Biological Psychiatry, 23*, 53–78. (9)

Morley, J. E., & Levine, A. S. (1980). Stress-induced eating is mediated through endogenous opiates. *Science, 209*, 1259–1261. (54)

Mormont, C., & Demoulin, C. (1971). La personnalité d'une anorexique mentale et de sa jumelle monozygote. *Acta Psychiatrica Belgium, 71*, 477–487. (89)

Morton, R. (1694). *Phthisiologia: Or a treatise of consumptions*. London: Smith & Walford. (2, 56)

Moskovitz, R. A., Belar, C., & Bingus, C. M. (1982). Anorexia nervosa in identical twins. *Hospital and Community Psychiatry, 33*, 484–485. (89)

Mumford, D. B., & Whitehouse, A. M. (1988). Increased prevalence of bulimia nervosa among Asian schoolgirls. *British Medical Journal, 297*, 718. (71)

Needleman, H. L., & Waber, D. (1977). Use of amitriptyline in anorexia nervosa. In R. Vigersky (Ed.), *Anorexia nervosa* (pp. 357–362). New York: Raven Press. (151)

Neil, J. F., Merikangas, J. R., Foster, F. G., Merikangas, K. R., Spiker, D. G., & Kupfer, D. J. (1980). Waking and all-night sleep EEG's in anorexia nervosa. *Clinical Electroencephalography, 11*, 9–15. (41)

Neki, J. S., Mohan, D., & Sood, R. K. (1977). Anorexia nervosa in a monozygotic twin pair. *Journal of the Indian Medical Association, 68*, 98–100. (89)

Nemiah, J. C. (1950). Anorexia nervosa. *Medicine, 29*, 225–268. (9, 37)

Nestel, P. J. (1973). Cholesterol metabolism in anorexia nervosa and hypercholesterolemia. *Journal of Clinical Endocrinology and Metabolism, 38*, 325–328. (41)

Nicolle, G. (1938). Pre-psychotic anorexia. *Lancet, ii*, 1173–1174. (8)

Nillius, S. J., & Wide, L. (1977). The pituitary responsiveness to acute and chronic administration of gonadotropin-releasing hormone in acute and recovery stages of anorexia nervosa. In R. A. Vigersky (Ed.), *Anorexia nervosa* (pp. 225–242). New York: Raven Press. (48)

Nogami, Y., & Yabana, F. (1977). On kibarashi-qui. *Folia Psychiatry Neurology Japan, 31*, 159–166. (4, 70)

Noles, S. W., Cash, T. F., & Winstead, B. A. (1985). Body image, physical attractiveness, and depression. *Journal of Consulting and Clinical Psychology, 53*, 88–94. (83)

Nowlin, N. (1983). Anorexia nervosa in twins: Case report and review. *Journal of Clinical Psychiatry, 44*, 101-105. (88)

Nussbaum, M., Shenker, I. R., Marc, J., & Klein, M. (1980). Cerebral atrophy in anorexia nervosa. *Journal of Pediatrics, 96*, 867-869. (42)

Nylander, I. (1971). The feeling of being fat and dieting in a school population: Epidemiologic interview investigation. *Acta Sociomedica Scandinavica, 3*, 17-26. (5, 67)

Offer, D., & Offer, J. B. (1975). *From teenage to young manhood: A psychological study.* New York: Basic Books. (82)

Ollendick, T. H. (1979). Behavior treatment of anorexia nervosa: A five-year study. *Behavior Modification, 3*, 124-135. (142)

Olson, D. H., Bell, R., & Protner, J. (1978). *Family adaptability and cohesion evaluation scale.* St. Paul, MN: Family Social Science, University of Minnesota. (38)

O'Mally, P. M., & Bachman, J. G. (1979). Self-esteem and education: Sex and cohort comparisons among high school seniors. *Journal of Personality and Social Psychology, 37*, 1153-1159. (82)

Orbach, S. (1985). Accepting the symptom: A feminist psychoanalytic treatment of anorexia nervosa. In D. M. Garner & P. E. Garfinkel (Eds.), *Handbook of psychotherapy for anorexia nervosa and bulimia* (pp. 83-106). New York: Guilford Press. (87, 106, 128)

Ordman, A. M., & Kirschenbaum, D. S. (1985). Cognitive–behavioral therapy for bulimia: An initial outcome study. *Journal of Consulting and Clinical Psychology, 53*, 305-313. (167)

Ordman, A. M., & Kirschenbaum, D. S. (1986). Bulimia: Assessment of eating, psychological adjustment, and familial characteristics. *International Journal of Eating Disorders, 5*, 865-878. (38)

Orlinsky, D. E., & Howard, K. I. (1986). Process and outcome in psychotherapy. In S. I. Garfield & A. E. Bergin (Eds.), *Handbook of psychotherapy and behavior change* (pp. 311-384). New York: Wiley. (126)

Orlofsky, J. L. (1978). Identity formation, need for achievement, and fear of success in college men and women. *Journal of Youth and Adolescence, 7*, 49-62. (86)

Palazzoli, M. S. (1978). *Self-starvation: From the intrapsychic to transpersonal approach.* New York: Jason Aronson. (28, 87, 126)

Palazzoli, M. S., Boscolo, L., Cecchin, G. C., & Prata, G. (1977). Family rituals: A powerful tool in family therapy. *Family Process, 16*, 445-453. (147)

Palazzoli, M. S., Boscolo, L., Cecchin, G., & Prata, G. (1980). Hypothesizing–circularity–neutrality: Three guidelines for the conductor of the session. *Family Process, 19*, 3-12. (149)

Palla, B., & Litt, I. F. (1988). Medical complications of eating disorders in adolescents. *Pediatrics, 81*, 613-623. (40)

Palmer, R. L. (1979). The dietary chaos syndrome: A useful new term? *British Journal of Medical Psychology, 52*, 187-190. (4)

Palmer, R. L., & Jones, M. S. (1939). Anorexia nervosa as a manifestation of compulsion neurosis. *Archives of Neurological Psychiatry, 41*, 856-861. (8)

Patton, G. C. (1988a). Mortality in eating disorders. *Psychological Medicine, 18,* 947–952. (192)

Patton, G. C. (1988b). The spectrum of eating disorder in adolescence. *Journal of Psychosomatic Research, 32,* 579–584. (5, 69, 83, 101, 161, 210)

Pemberton, C. M., & Gastineau, C. F. (1981). *Mayo clinic diet manual: A handbook of dietary practices* (5th ed., pp. 114–117). Philadelphia: W. B. Saunders. (162)

Pfeiffer, R. J., Lucas, A. R., & Ilstrup, D. M. (1986). Effect of anorexia nervosa on linear growth. *Clinical Pediatrics, 25,* 7–12. (40)

Pillay, M., & Crisp, A. H. (1981). The impact of social skills training for anorexia nervosa. *British Journal of Psychiatry, 139,* 533–539. (142)

Piran, N., Kennedy, S., Garfinkel, P. E., & Owens, M. (1985). Affective disturbance in eating disorders. *Journal of Nervous and Mental Disease, 173,* 395–400. (10)

Pirke, K. M., Pahl, J., Schweiger, U., & Warnhoff, M. (1985). Metabolic and endocrine indices of starvation in bulimia: A comparison with anorexia nervosa. *Psychiatry Research, 15,* 33–39. (10, 41)

Pirke, K. M., Schweiger, U., & Fichter, M. M. (1987). Hypothalamic–pituitary–ovarian axis in bulimia. In J. I. Hudson & H. G. Pope (Eds.), *The psychobiology of bulimia* (pp. 15–28). Washington, DC: American Psychiatric Press. (26)

Pirke, K. M., Schweiger, U., Laessle, R., Fichter, M. M., & Wolfram, G. (1987). Metabolic and endocrine consequences of eating behavior and food composition in bulimia. In J. I. Hudson & H. G. Pope (Eds.). *The psychobiology of bulimia* (pp. 131–143). Washington, DC: American Psychiatric Press. (24)

Polivy, J., & Herman, C. P. (1976). Clinical depression and weight change: A complex relation. *Journal of Abnormal Psychology, 85,* 338–340. (97)

Polivy, J., Herman, C. P., Olmsted, M. P., & Jazwinski, C. (1984). Restraint and binge eating. In R. C. Hawkins, W. J. Fremouw, & P. F. Clement (Eds.), *The binge–purge syndrome: Diagnosis, treatment and research* (pp. 104–122). New York: Springer. (161)

Pope, H. G., Jr., Frankenburg, F. R., Hudson, J. I., Jonas, J. M., & Yurgelun-Todd, D. (1987). Is bulimia associated with borderline personality disorder? A controlled study. *Journal of Clinical Psychiatry, 48,* 181–184. (30, 97)

Pope, H. G., Jr., & Hudson, J. I. (1982). Treatment of bulimia with antidepressants. *Psychopharmacology, 78,* 176–179. (175)

Pope, H. G., Jr., & Hudson, J. I. (1988). Is bulimia nervosa a heterogeneous disorder? Lessons from the history of medicine. *International Journal of Eating Disorders, 7,* 155–166. (9)

Pope, H. G., Jr., Hudson, J. I., Jonas, J. M., & Yurgelun-Todd, D. (1983). Bulimia treated with imipramine: A placebo-controlled, double-blind study. *American Journal of Psychiatry, 140,* 554–558. (175)

Pope, H. G., Jr., Hudson, J. I., & Mialet, J. P. (1985). Bulimia in the late nineteenth century: The observations of Pierre Janet. *Psychological Medicine, 15,* 739–743. (4)

Pope, H. G., Jr., Hudson, J. I., & Yurgelun-Todd, D. (1984). Anorexia nervosa and bulimia among 300 suburban women shoppers. *American Journal of Psychiatry, 141,* 292-294. (67)

Post, F. (1972). The management and nature of depressive illnesses in late life: A follow through study. *British Journal of Psychiatry, 121,* 393-404. (11)

Powers, P. S., & Powers, H. P. (1984). Inpatient treatment of anorexia nervosa. *Psychosomatics, 25,* 512-527. (137)

Pumariega, A. J. (1986). Acculturation and eating attitudes in adolescent girls: A comparative and correctional study. *Journal of the American Academy of Child Psychiatry, 25,* 276-279. (80)

Pyle, R. L., Halvorson, P. A., Neuman, P. A., & Mitchell, J. E. (1986). The increasing prevalence of bulimia in freshman college students. *International Journal of Eating Disorders, 5,* 631-647. (70)

Pyle, R. L., Mitchell, J. E., & Eckert, E. D. (1981). Bulimia: A report of 34 cases. *Journal of Clinical Psychiatry, 42,* 60-64. (160)

Pyle, R. L., Mitchell, J. E., Eckert, E. D., Halvorson, P. A., Neuman, P. A., & Goff, G. M. (1983). The incidence of bulimia in freshman college students. *International Journal of Eating Disorders, 2,* 75-85. (21, 67)

Rahman, L., Richardson, H. B., & Ripley, H. S. (1939). Anorexia nervosa with psychiatric observations. *Psychosomatic Medicine, 1,* 335-365. (8)

Rainer, J. D. (1982). Genetics of schizophrenia. In J. K. Wing & L. Wing (Eds.), *Handbook of psychiatry* (Vol. 3, pp. 62-67). Cambridge: Cambridge University Press. (88)

Rampling, D. (1978). Anorexia nervosa: Reflections on theory and practice. *Psychiatry, 41,* 296-301. (126)

Rampling, D. (1980). Abnormal mothering in the genesis of anorexia nervosa. *Journal of Nervous and Mental Disorders, 168,* 501-504. (100)

Rau, J. H., & Green, R. S. (1984). Neurological factors affecting binge eating: Body over mind. In R. C. Hawkins, W. J. Fremouw, & P. F. Clement (Eds.), *The binge-purge syndrome: Diagnosis, treatment, and research* (pp. 123-143). New York: Springer. (42, 179)

Reed, D. R., Contreras, R. J., Maggio, C., Greenwood, M. R. C., & Rodin, J. (1988). Weight cycling in female rats increases dietary fat selection and adiposity. *Physiology and Behavior, 42,* 389-395. (211)

Reinhart, J. B., Kenna, M. D., & Succop, R. A. (1972). Anorexia nervosa in children: Outpatient management. *Journal of the American Academy of Child Psychiatry, 11,* 114-131. (132)

Rich, C. L. (1978). Self-induced vomiting: Psychiatric considerations. *Journal of the American Medical Association, 239,* 2688-2689. (175)

Rigotti, N. A., Nussbaum, S. R., Herzog, D. B., & Neer, R. M. (1984). Osteoporosis in women with anorexia nervosa. *New England Journal of Medicine, 311,* 1601-1606. (40)

Rivinis, T. M., Biederman, J., Herzog, D. B., Kemper, K., Harper, G. P., Harmatz, J. S., & Houseworth, S. (1984). Anorexia nervosa and affective disorder: A controlled family history. *American Journal of Psychiatry, 141,* 1414-1418. (35)

Robinson, P. H., Checkley, S. A., & Russell, G. F. M. (1985). Suppression of eating by fenfluramine in patients with bulimia nervosa. *British Journal of Psychiatry, 146,* 169-176. (180)

Roden, J., Silberstein, L. R., & Steigel-Moore, R. H. (1985). Women and weight: A normative discontent. In T. B. Sonderegger (Ed.), *Nebraska symposium on motivation: Vol. 32. Psychology and gender* (pp. 267-307). Lincoln: University of Nebraska. (79)

Root, M. P. P., Fallon, P., & Friedrich, W. N. (1986). *Bulimia: A systems approach to treatment.* New York: Norton. (174)

Rosen, L. W., & Hough, D. O. (1988). Pathogenic weight-control behaviors of female college athletes. *Physician in Sports Medicine, 16,* 141-146. (72)

Rosen, J. C., & Leitenberg, H. (1982). Bulimia nervosa: Treatment with exposure and response prevention. *Behavior Therapy, 13,* 117-124. (97, 163)

Rosen, J. C., & Leitenberg, H. (1985). Exposure plus response prevention treatment for bulimia. In D. M. Garner & P. E. Garfinkel (Eds.), *Handbook of psychotherapy for anorexia nervosa and bulimia* (pp. 193-209). New York: Guilford Press. (169)

Rosen, J. C., Leitenberg, H., Fisher, C., & Khazam, C. (1986). Binge-eating episodes in bulimia nervosa: The amount and type of food consumed. *International Journal of Eating Disorders, 5,* 255-268. (21)

Rosman, B. L., Minuchin, S., Baker, L., & Liebman, R. (1977). A family approach to anorexia nervosa: Study, treatment, and outcome. In R. A. Vigersky (Ed.), *Anorexia nervosa* (pp. 341-348). New York: Raven Press. (149, 187)

Rothenberg, A. (1986). Eating disorder as a modern obsessive–compulsive syndrome. *Psychiatry, 49,* 45-53. (8)

Roy-Bryne, P., Lee-Benner, K., & Yager, J. (1984). Group therapy for bulimia: A year's experience. *International Journal of Eating Disorders, 3,* 97-116. (161)

Russell, G. F. M. (1970). Anorexia nervosa: Its identity as an illness and its treatment. In J. H. Price (Ed.), *Modern trends in psychological medicine* (Vol. 2, pp. 131-164). London: Butterworths. (3, 61, 98, 115, 135, 188)

Russell, G. F. M. (1977a). The present status of anorexia nervosa. *Psychological Medicine, 7,* 353-367. (26, 98)

Russell, G. F. M. (1977b). General management of anorexia nervosa and difficulties in assessing the efficacy of treatment. In R. A. Vigersky (Ed.), *Anorexia nervosa* (pp. 277-290). New York: Raven. (131, 189)

Russell, G. F. M. (1979). Bulimia nervosa: An ominous variant of anorexia nervosa. *Psychological Medicine, 9,* 429-448. (4, 16, 116, 157, 207)

Russell, G. F. M. (1985). The changing nature of anorexia nervosa: An introduction to the conference. *Journal of Psychiatric Resaerch, 19,* 101-109. (7, 98, 116)

Russell, G. F. M., Checkley, S. A., Feldman, J., & Eisler, I. (1988). A controlled trial of d-fenfluramine in bulimia nervosa. *Clinical Neuropharmacology, 11*(Suppl. 1), 146-159. (180)

Russell, G. F. M., Szmukler, G. I., Dare, C., & Eisler, I. (1987). An evaluation of family therapy in anorexia nervosa and bulimia nervosa. *Archives of General Psychiatry, 44,* 1047-1056. (149, 201)

Rutter, M., Cox, A., Tupling, C., Berger, M., & Yule, W. (1975). Attainment and adjustment in two geographical areas. I. The prevalence of psychiatric disorders. *British Journal of Psychiatry, 126,* 493–509. (82)

Rutter, M., Graham, P., Chadwick, O., & Yule, W. (1976). Adolescent turmoil: Fact or fiction. *Journal of Child Psychology and Psychiatry, 17,* 35–56. (82)

Salkind, M. R., Fincham, J., & Silverstone, T. (1980). Is anorexia nervosa a phobic disorder? *Biological Psychiatry, 15,* 803–809. (96)

Sanger, D. J. (1981). Endorphinergic mechanisms in the control of food and water intake. *Appetite: Journal of Intake Research, 2,* 193–208. (54)

Sargent, J., Liebman, R., & Silver, M. (1985). Family therapy for anorexia nervosa. In D. M. Garner & P. E. Garfinkel (Eds.), *Handbook of psychotherapy for anorexia nervosa and bulimia* (pp. 257–279). New York: Guilford Press. (100, 125)

Savin-Williams, R. (1979). Dominance hierarchies in groups of early adolescents. *Child Development, 50,* 923–935. (82)

Schiele, B. C., & Brozek, J. (1948). Experimental neurosis resulting from semistarvation in man. *Psychosomatic Medicine, 10,* 31–50. (17)

Schneider, J. A., & Agras, W. S. (1985). A cognitive–behavioral group treatment of bulimia. *British Journal of Psychiatry, 146,* 66–69. (170)

Schneider, J. A., & Agras, W. S. (1987). Bulimia in males: A matched comparison with females. *International Journal of Eating Disorders, 6,* 235–242. (57)

Schnurer, A. T., Rubin, R. R., & Roy, A. (1973). Systematic desensitization of anorexia nervosa seen as a weight phobia. *Journal of Behavior Therapy and Experimental Psychiatry, 4,* 149–153. (142)

Schwartz, R. C., Barrett, M. J., & Saba, G. (1985). Family therapy for bulimia. In D. M. Garner & P. E. Garfinkel (Eds.), *Handbook of psychotherapy for anorexia nervosa and bulimia* (pp. 280–307). New York: Guilford Press. (174)

Scott, D. W. (1987). Anorexia nervosa in the male: A review of clinical epidemiological and biological findings. *International Journal of Eating Disorders, 5,* 799–820. (57)

Seidensticker, J. F., & Tzagournis, M. (1968). Anorexia nervosa: Clinical features and long-term follow-up. *Journal of Chronic Diseases, 21,* 361–367. (11, 187)

Sheehan, H. L., & Summers, V. K. (1949). The syndrome of hypopituitarism. *Quarterly Journal of Medicine, 18,* 319–378. (2)

Silverman, J. A. (1977). Anorexia nervosa: Clinical and metabolic observations in a successful treatment plan. In R. A. Vigersky (Ed.), *Anorexia nervosa* (pp. 331–340). New York: Raven. (187)

Silverman, J. A. (1983). Anorexia nervosa: Clinical and metabolic observations. *International Journal of Eating Disorders, 2,* 159–166. (40)

Silverstone, J. T., Gordon, R. A. P., & Stunkard, A. J. (1969). Social factors in obesity in London. *The Practitioner, 202,* 682–688. (79)

Simmonds, M. (1914). Ueber embolische prozesse in der hypophysis. *Archiv fur Pathologie und Anatomie, 217,* 226–239. (2)

Simmons, R. G., Blyth, D. A., & McKinney, K. L. (1983). The social and psychological effects on white females. In J. Brooks-Gunn & A. C. Petersen (Eds.), *Girls at puberty* (pp. 229–272). New York: Plenum Press. (84)

Simmons, R. G., & Kessler, M. D. (1979). Identical twins simultaneously concordant for anorexia nervosa. *Journal of the American Academy of Child Psychiatry, 18*, 527-536. (89)

Simmons, R. G., & Rosenberg, F. (1975). Sex, sex roles, and image. *Journal of Youth and Adolescence, 4*, 229-258. (82)

Singer, J. E., & Lamb, P. F. (1966). Social concern, body size, and birth order. *Journal of Social Psychology, 68*, 143-151. (79)

Slade, P. (1982). Towards a functional analysis of anorexia nervosa and bulimia nervosa. *British Journal of Clinical Psychology, 21*, 167-179. (97)

Smart, D. E., Beumont, P. J. V., & George, G. C. W. (1976). Some personality characteristics of patients with anorexia nervosa. *British Journal of Psychiatry, 128*, 57-60. (28)

Society of Actuaries and Association of Life Insurance Medical Directors of America (1979). *Build and Blood Pressure Study.* Chicago, IL: Author. (78)

Sonne-Holm, S., & Sorensen, T. I. A. (1977). Post-war course of the prevalence of extreme overweight among Danish young men. *Journal of Chronic Disease, 30*, 351-358. (78)

Sours, J. A. (Ed.). (1980). *Starving to death in a sea of objects.* New York: Jason Aronson. (29, 96, 143)

Spitzer, R. L., Williams, J. B. W., Gibbon, M., & First, M. B. (1988). *The structured clinical interview for DSM-III-R, non-patient version.* New York: Biometrics Research Department, New York State Psychiatric Institute. (110)

Staffieri, J. R. (1967). A study of social stereotype of body image in children. *Journal of Personality and Social Psychology, 7*, 101-104. (84)

Steinhausen, H. C., & Glanville, K. (1983). A long-term follow-up of adolescent anorexia nervosa. *Acta Psychiatrica Scandinavica, 68*, 1-10. (187)

Stern, S. L., Dixon, K. N., Nemzer, E., Lake, M. D., Sansone, R. A., Smeltzer, D. J., Lantz, S., & Schrier, S. S. (1984). Affective disorder in the families of women with normal weight bulimia. *American Journal of Psychiatry, 141*, 1224-1227. (35)

Stordy, B. J., Marks, V., Kalucy, R. S., & Crisp, A. H. (1977). Weight gain, thermic effect of glucose and resting metabolic rate during recovery from anorexia nervosa. *American Journal of Clinical Nutrition, 30*, 138-146. (28)

Strober, M. (1980). Personality and symptomatological features in young, non-chronic anorexia nervosa patients. *Journal of Psychosomatic Research, 24*, 353-359. (28)

Strober, M. (1981). A comparative analysis of personality organization in juvenile anorexia nervosa. *Journal of Youth and Adolescence, 10*, 285-295. (28, 94)

Strober, M. (1984). Stressful life events associated with bulimia in anorexia nervosa: Empirical findings and theoretical speculations. *International Journal of Eating Disorders, 3*, 3-16. (23)

Strober, M., & Katz, J. L. (1987). Do eating disorders and affective disorders share a common etiology? *International Journal of Eating Disorders, 6*, 171-180. (9, 205)

Strober, M., & Katz, J. L. (1988). Depression in eating disorders: A review and analysis of descriptive, family, and biological findings. In D. M. Garner &

P. E. Garfinkel (Eds.), *Diagnostic issues in anorexia nervosa and bulimia nervosa* (pp. 80-111). New York: Brunner/Mazel. (36)

Strober, M., Morrell, W., Burroughs, J., Salkin, B., & Jacobs, C. (1985). A controlled family study of anorexia nervosa. *Journal of Psychiatric Research, 19*, 239-246. (7, 33)

Strober, M., Salkin, B., Burroughs, J., & Morrell, W. (1982). Validity of the bulimia-restrictor distinction in anorexia nervosa. *Journal of Nervous and Mental Disease, 170*, 345-351. (36, 95)

Strober, M., & Yager, J. (1985). A developmental perspective on the treatment of anorexia nervosa in adolescents. In D. M. Garner & P. E. Garfinkel (Eds.), *Handbook of psychotherapy for anorexia nervosa and bulimia* (pp. 363-390). New York: Guilford Press. (125)

Stunkard, A. J. (1959). Eating patterns and obesity. *Psychiatric Quarterly, 33*, 284-292. (4, 181)

Stunkard, A. J. (1977). Obesity and the social environment: Current status, future prospects. *Proceedings of the New York Academy of Sciences, 300*, 298-320. (78)

Sturzenberger, S., Cantwell, D., Burroughs, J., Salkin, B., & Green, J. (1977). A follow-up study of adolescent psychiatric inpatients with anorexia nervosa. *Journal of the American Academy of Child Psychiatry, 16*, 703-715. (188)

Styczynsi, L., & Langlois, J. H. (1977). The effects of familiarity on behavioral stereotypes associated with physical attractiveness in young children. *Child Development, 48*, 1137-1141. (84)

Suematsu, H., Ishikawa, H., Kubocki, T., & Ito, T. (1985). Statistical studies on anorexia nervosa in Japan: Detailed clinical data on 1011 patients. *Psychotherapy and Psychosomatics, 43*, 96-103. (70)

Swift, W. J., Kalin, N. H., Wamboldt, F. S., Kaslow, N., & Ritholz, M. (1985). Depression in bulimia at 2- to 5-year follow-up. *Psychiatric Research, 16*, 111-122. (9)

Swift, W. J., Ritholz, M., Kalin, N. H., & Kaslow, N. (1987). A follow-up study of thirty hospitalized bulimics. *Psychosomatic Medicine, 49*, 45-55. (10, 201)

Sydenham, A. (1946). Amenorrhoea at Stanley Camp, Hong Kong during internment. *British Medical Journal, ii*, 159. (25)

Szmukler, G. I. (1983). Weight and food preoccupation in a population of English schoolgirls. In G. J. Bargman (Ed.), *Understanding anorexia nervosa and bulimia* (pp. 21-27) (Fourth Ross Conference on Medical Research). Columbus, OH: Ross Laboratories. (65)

Szmukler, G. I. (1985). The epidemiology of anorexia nervosa and bulimia. *Journal of Psychiatric Research, 19*, 143-153. (60, 198)

Szmukler, G. I., Eisler, I., Gillis, C., & Hayward, M. E. (1985). The implications of anorexia nervosa in a ballet school. *Journal of Psychiatric Research, 19*, 177-181. (5, 61, 161)

Szmukler, G. I., McCance, C., McCrone, L., & Hunter, D. (1986). A psychiatric case register study from Aberdeen. *Psychological Medicine, 16*, 49-58. (62)

Szyrynski, V. (1973). Anorexia nervosa and psychotherapy. *American Journal of Psychotherapy, 27*, 492-505. (61, 126)

Taylor, M. J., & Cooper, P. J. (1986). Body size overestimation and depressed mood. *British Journal of Clinical Psychology, 25*, 153–154. (83)

Theander, S. (1970). Anorexia nervosa: A psychiatric investigation of 94 female patients. *Acta Psychiatrica Scandinavica,* (Suppl. 214), 1–194. (23, 61, 192)

Theander, S. (1985). Outcome and prognosis in anorexia nervosa and bulimia: Some results of previous investigations, compared with those of a Swedish long-term study. *Journal of Psychiatric Research, 19*, 493–508. (194)

Thoma, H. (1967). *Anorexia nervosa.* New York: International Universities Press. (187)

Tinker, D. E., & Ramer, J. C. (1983). Anorexia nervosa: Staff subversion of therapy. *Journal of Adolescent Health Care, 4*, 35–39. (133)

Tobin-Richards, M. H., Boxer, A. M., & Petersen, A. C. (1983). The psychological significance of pubertal change. Sex differences in perceptions of self during early adolescence. In J. Brooks-Gunn & A. C. Petersen (Eds.), *Girls at puberty* (pp. 127–154). New York: Plenum Press. (82)

Toner, B. B., Garfinkel, P. E., & Garner, D. M. (1986). Long-term follow-up of anorexia nervosa. *Psychosomatic Medicine, 48*, 520–529. (191)

Touyz, S. W., Beumont, P. J. V., & Glaun, D. (1984). A comparison of lenient and strict operant conditioning in refeeding patients with anorexia nervosa. *British Journal of Psychiatry, 144*, 517–520. (141)

Treasure, J. L. (1988). The ultrasonographic features in anorexia nervosa and bulimia nervosa: A simplified method of monitoring hormonal states during weight gain. *Journal of Psychosomatic Research, 32*, 624–634. (25)

Treasure, J. L., & Russell, G. F. M. (1988). Intrauterine growth and neonatal weight gain in anorexia nervosa. *British Medical Journal, 296*, 1038. (197)

Treasure, J. L., Russell, G. F. M., Fogelman, I., & Murby, B. (1987). Reversible bone loss in anorexia nervosa. *British Medical Journal, 295*, 474–475. (40)

Valanne, E. H., Tiapale, V., Larkio-Miettinen, A. K., Moren, R., & Aukee, M. (1972). Anorexia nervosa: A follow-up study. *Psychiatria Fennica,* 265–269. (188)

Vandereycken, W. (1984). Neuroleptics in the short-term treatment of anorexia nervosa. A double-blind, placebo-controlled study with sulpiride. *British Journal of Psychiatry, 144*, 288–292. (151)

Vandereycken, W. (1987). The use of neuroleptics in the treatment of anorexia nervosa patients. In P. E. Garfinkel & D. M. Garner (Eds.), *The role of drug treatments for eating disorders* (pp. 74–89). New York: Brunner/Mazel. (54, 152)

Vandereycken, W., & Meermann, R. (1984). Anorexia nervosa: Is prevention possible? *International Journal of Psychiatry in Medicine, 14*, 191–205. (210)

Vandereycken, W., & Pierloot, R. (1982). Pimozide combined with behavior therapy in the short-term treatment of anorexia nervosa: A double-blind, placebo-controlled cross-over study. *Acta Psychiatrica Scandinavica, 66*, 445–450. (151)

Vigersky, R. A., & Loriaux, D. L. (1977). Anorexia nervosa as a model of hypothalamic dysfunction. In R. A. Vigersky (Ed.), *Anorexia nervosa* (pp. 109–122). New York: Raven Press. (151)

Wakeling, A. (1985). Neurobiological aspects of feeding disorders. *Journal of Psychiatric Research, 19*, 191–201. (48)

Wakeling, A., DeSouza, V. A., & Beardwood, C. J. (1977). Assessment of negative and positive feedback effects of administered oestrogen on gonadotrophin release in patients with anorexia nervosa. *Psychological Medicine, 7*, 397–405. (26)

Wall, J. H. (1959). Diagnosis, treatment and results in anorexia nervosa. *American Journal of Psychiatry, 115*, 997–1001. (27)

Waller, J., Kaufman, M. R., & Deutsch, F. (1940). Anorexia nervosa: A psychosomatic study. *Psychosomatic Medicine, 2*, 3–16. (96)

Walsh, B. T. (1982). Endocrine disturbances in anorexia nervosa and depression. *Psychosomatic Medicine, 44*, 85–91. (48)

Walsh, B. T., Goetz, R., Roose, S. P., Fingeroth, S., & Glassman, A. H. (1985). EEG-monitored sleep in anorexia nervosa and bulimia. *Biological Psychiatry, 20*, 947–956. (42)

Walsh, B. T., Kissileff, H. R., Cassidy, S. M., & Dantzic, S. (1989). Eating behavior of women with bulimia. *Archives of General Psychiatry, 46*, 54–58. (21)

Walsh, B. T., Roose, S. P., Glassman, A. H., Gladis, M., & Sadik, C. (1985). Bulimia and depression. *Psychosomatic Medicine, 47*, 123–131. (9)

Walsh, B. T., Roose, S. P., Lindy, D. C., Gladis, M., & Glassman, A. H. (1987). Hypothalamic–pituitary–adrenal axis in bulimia. In J. I. Hudson & H. G. Pope (Eds.), *The psychobiology of bulimia* (pp. 3–11). Washington, DC: American Psychiatric Press. (55)

Walsh, B. T., Stewart, J. W., Roose, S. P., Gladis, M., & Glassman, A. H. (1984). Treatment of bulimia with phenelzine: A double-blind, placebo-controlled study. *Archives of General Psychiatry, 41*, 1105–1109. (177)

Walsh, B. T., Stewart, J. W., Wright, L., Harrison, W., Roose, S. P., & Glassman, A. H. (1982). Treatment of bulimia with monoamine oxidase inhibitors. *American Journal of Psychiatry, 129*, 1629–1630. (175)

Walster, E., Aronson, V., Abrahams, D., & Rottman, L. (1966). Importance of physical attractiveness in dating behavior. *Journal of Personality and Social Psychology, 4*, 508–516. (84)

Wardle, J., & Beales, S. (1986). Restraint, body image and food attitudes in children from 12 to 18 years. *Appetite, 7*, 209–217. (80)

Warren, M. P. (1977). Weight loss and responsiveness to LH-RH. In R. A. Vigersky (Ed.), *Anorexia nervosa* (pp. 189–198). New York: Raven. (49)

Warren, W. (1968). A study of anorexia nervosa in young girls. *Journal of Child Psychology and Psychiatry and Allied Disciplines, 9*, 27–40. (11)

Watson, D., & Friend, R. (1969). Measurement of social evaluative anxiety. *Journal of Consulting and Clinical Psychology, 33*, 448–457. (122)

Weiner, H. (1983). The hypothalamic–pituitary–ovarian axis in anorexia and bulimia nervosa. *International Journal of Eating Disorders, 2*, 109–116. (48)

Weiner, J. M. (1976). Identical male twins discordant for anorexia nervosa. *Journal of the American Academy of Child Psychiatry, 15*, 523–534. (89)

Weiss, S. R., & Ebert, M. H. (1983). Psychological and behavioral characteristics of normal weight bulimics. *Psychosomatic Medicine, 45*, 293–303. (24)

Weiss, L., Katzman, M., & Wolchik, S. (1985). *Treating bulimia: A psychoeducational approach.* New York: Pergamon Press. (182)

Weller, R. A., & Weller, E. B. (1982). Anorexia nervosa in a patient with an infiltrating tumor of the hypothalamus. *American Journal of Psychiatry, 139*, 824–825. (40)

Wermuth, B. M., Davis, K. L., Hollister, L. E., & Stunkard, A. J. (1977). Phenytoin treatment of the binge-eating syndrome. *American Journal of Psychiatry*, *134*, 1249-1253. (177)

Whitehouse, A. M., & Button, E. J. (1988). The prevalence of eating disorders in a U.K. college population: A reclassification of an earlier study. *International Journal of Eating Disorders*, *7*, 393-397. (68)

Willi, J., & Grossman, S. (1983). Epidemiology of anorexia nervosa in a defined region of Switzerland. *American Journal of Psychiatry*, *140*, 564-567. (61)

Williams, E. (1958). Anorexia nervosa: A somatic disorder. *British Medical Journal*, *ii*, 190-194. (131, 189)

Williams, P., Hand, D., & Tarnopolsky, A. (1982). The problem of screening for uncommon disorders—A comment on the eating attitudes test. *Psychological Medicine*, *12*, 431-434. (65)

Williams, P., Tarnopolsky, A., & Hand, D. (1980). Case definition and case identification in psychiatric epidemiology: Review and assessment. *Psychological Medicine*, *10*, 101-114. (65)

Wilson, C. P. (1983). The fear of being fat in female psychology. In C. P. Wilson (Ed.), *Fear of being fat* (pp. 9-27). New York: Jason Aronson. (131)

Wilson, G. T., Rossiter, E., Kleifeld, E. L., & Lindholm, L. (1986). Cognitive-behavioral treatment of bulimia nervosa: A controlled evaluation. *Behavior Research and Therapy*, *24*, 277-288. (167, 201)

Wilson, A. J., Touyz, S. W., O'Connor, M., & Beumont, P. J. V. (1985). Correcting the eating disorder in anorexia nervosa. *Journal of Psychiatric Research*, *19*, 449-451. (139)

Winokur, A., March, V., & Mendels, J. (1980). Primary affective disorder in relatives of patients with anorexia nervosa. *American Journal of Psychiatry*, *137*, 695-698. (35)

Wolchik, S. A., Weiss, L., & Katzman, M. A. (1986). An empirical validated short-term psychoeducational group treatment program for bulimia. *International Journal of Eating Disorders*, *5*, 21-34. (161)

Wooley, S. C., & Wooley, O. W. (1985). Intensive outpatient and residential treatment for bulimia. In D. M. Garner & P. E. Garfinkel (Eds.), *Handbook of psychotherapy for anorexia nervosa* (pp. 391-430). New York: Guilford Press. (146)

Yager, J. (1982). Family issues in the pathogenesis of anorexia nervosa. *Psychosomatic Medicine*, *44*, 43-60. (99)

Yager, J., Landsverk, J., & Edelstein, C. K. (1987). A 20-month follow-up study of 628 women with eating disorders. I: Course and severity. *American Journal of Psychiatry*, *144*, 1172-1177. (161, 201)

Yates, A., Leehey, K., & Shisslak, C. M. (1983). Running—An analogue of anorexia? *The New England Journal of Medicine*, *308*, 252-255. (72)

Zohar, J., Insel, T. R., Zohar-Kadouh, R. C., Hill, J. L., & Murphy, D. L. (1988). Serotonin function in obsessive-compulsive disorder. *Archives of General Psychiatry*, *45*, 167-172. (9)

Index